MW00658485

A Quiet World

A Quiet World

Living with Hearing Loss

DAVID G. MYERS

Yale University Press New Haven and London

Published with assistance from the Williams Memorial Fund.

Designed by James J. Johnson and set in Stemple Garamond types by The Composing Room of Michigan, Inc.
Printed in the United States of America by Sheridan Books, Chelsea, Michigan.

Library of Congress Catologing-in-Publication Data

Myers, David G.
A quiet world : living with hearing loss / David G. Myers.
p. cm.
Includes index.
ISBN 978-0-300-19465-4

1. Deafness—Popular works. 2. Hearing disorders—Popular works. 3. Hearing aids. I. Title.
RF290 .M84 2000
617.8—dc21 00-038153
A catalogue record for this book is available from the British Library.

The paper in this book meets the guidelines for permanence and durability of the Committee on Production Guidelines for Book Longevity of the Council on Library Resources.

10 9 8 7 6 5 4 3 2 1

To the memory of

Luella Nelson Myers,

whose journey from sound to silence
I am coming to understand,

and to

Carol,

my supportive partner

Contents

Preface

Some 28 million Americans and 350 million people worldwide live with hearing loss. What is it like? How do those who are hard of hearing cope? What are their experiences of pain and pathos, of hope and humor? How can medicine and technology now assist people who are hard of hearing, and what is on the horizon?

This book offers some answers. My perspective combines my vocation as a research psychologist and writer with my experiences as the son of a woman deafened late in life and as a hard of hearing person. This unusual combination, it occurred to me one day, positioned me to speak about hearing, hearing loss, and hearing interventions as both a participant and an observer. To personalize the information, I have cast it in the form of an occasional journal in which I record both my experiences and, especially in the later entries, my encounters with new technologies and new insights into the nature of hearing.

While writing, I have imagined two audiences looking over my shoulder. The first is my peers, the hard of hearing—a fast-growing group because of the aging of our population and the cumulative effects of amplified music, power mowers, motorcycles, and blow dryers. As you read, I hope you will be stimulated to reflect on your experiences and on your own identity as a person with hearing loss.

My second audience is our loved ones. Here in America, that includes our more than 15 million spouses, 50 million or so children, and as many close friends. Sometimes, out of curiosity or exasperation, you wonder about our experience—what it sounds like, what it feels like. At other times, you wonder how best to alert us to hearing problems and persuade us to seek assistance. Drawing on both psychological research and my own experience, I hope first to help you understand the sometimes painful, sometimes hilarious experiences of hearing loss, and second to suggest how you might more effectively offer love and advice. Along the way we'll meet others who are living with hearing loss. And we will marvel at the intricacies of hearing and find hope in the latest hearing-assistive technology.

I am indebted to many for their support for this project. My poet-colleague Nancy Nicodemus inspired me to begin recording my experiences. My audiologist, Edward Szumowski, endured, and even led me to think he enjoyed, my endless questioning. Ear surgeon Michael Disher gave me additional information and directed me to the resources of Self Help for Hard of Hearing People. Susan Arellano at Yale University Press, sensitized by her belonging to one of the target audiences, comprehended and then helped shape my vision for this book. Letha Dawson Scanzoni provided both skilled editing and heartening encouragement, as did Susan Abel of Yale University Press at a later stage. The first four, along with a number of friends and family members, read early drafts and encouraged me to keep writing. Among those family members are my father, Kenneth, and my soul mate, Carol, who is sometimes my ears, sometimes my counselor, and sometimes my critic. To each of these, I offer my thanks.

1

Adaptation

From Sound to Silence

5 AUGUST 1990

On one of those treasured visits to my parents' home on Bainbridge Island, Washington, I use a magic pad to communicate with my eighty-year-old mother, who four years previously took the final step from hearing-impaired to deaf as she gave up wearing her by then useless hearing aids.

"Do you hear anything?" I write.

"No," she answers, her voice still strong although she cannot hear it. "Last night your Dad came in and found the T.V. blasting. Someone had left the volume way up; I didn't hear a thing." (Indeed, my father later explained, he recently tested her by sneaking up while she was reading and giving a loud clap just behind her ear. Her eye never wavered from the page.)

What is it like, I wonder. "A silent world?"

"Yes," she replies, "it's a silent world."

As with Mother, so, I expect, with me. I have known for many years that I am on a trajectory toward the same deafness. When tested as a teenager, my hearing pattern mimicked Mother's—an unusual "reverse slope" pattern of good hearing for high-pitched sounds and poorer hearing for low-pitched sounds (making soft male voices harder to discern than higher female voices). From upstairs, I can hear the high-pitched microwave oven timer, though my wife, Carol, snuggled beside me in bed, cannot. But I cannot recall ever hearing an owl hoot. Carol touches my leg at each hoot: "There, can you hear it?" I hear nothing.

When I was a graduate student, my peculiar hearing loss made me a case for study and discussion in front of twenty doctors and residents at the University of Iowa Medical School's hearing clinic. It was a foretaste of what Dr. Seuss predicted in *You're Only Old Once!*

> You'll be told that your hearing's so murky and muddy,
> your case calls for special intensified study.
> They'll test you with noises from far and from near
> and you'll get a black mark for the ones you can't hear.
> Then they'll say, "My dear fellow, you're deafer than most.
> But there's hope, since you're not quite as deaf as a post."

In my early forties, an audiologist (a specialist in assessing and alleviating hearing loss) wondered aloud how I was able to cope with life without a hearing aid. But my coping is far from perfect. Already, at forty-seven, I seek seats front and center at lectures, meetings, and the theater. In restaurants, I prefer corners or a seat against the wall. In the psychology classes I teach at Hope College in Michigan, students occasionally snicker when I answer a question inappropriately. At home, I sometimes miss what my children say. On visits to Scotland, I ask Carol to handle telephone calls; she can better discern words spoken with a brogue.

At the moment I have a 1980s-vintage hearing aid, but it magnifies all sounds—including those high-pitched sounds which I hear reasonably well. The clash of silverware becomes distracting, irritating, almost painfully loud. Part of that "loudness" may be relative to my adaptation to a quiet world, rather like the sun's seeming brightness that we complain about when we emerge from a movie. Bothersome loudness also results from a common but little-known oddity of hearing loss. Damaged hair-cell receptors within the inner ear may fail to respond to soft sounds yet respond normally to loud sounds (with a boost from neighboring hair cells that also begin to respond). Normal hearing progresses through sounds that range from quiet to moderate to loud and very loud. But once a person with significant loss *is* able to hear something, increasing loudness all too quickly becomes *very* loud and then uncomfortably loud. A person with hearing loss may therefore miss soft sounds that others hear but hear loud sounds quite normally. When all sounds—including loud sounds—are amplified, some noises are uncomfortably loud. (One doesn't need a hearing aid at a rock concert—an event that the hard of hearing will want to avoid anyway, to protect the inner ear's remaining healthy sensory receptors, the hair cells.)

Moreover, merely magnifying sound far from its source hardly improves its clarity. It's like a microphone recording a speaker from across a room: it records the reverberations of the voice and all the intervening sounds as well. You also have to put up with the distracting sound of your own distorted voice. So I seldom wear my hearing aid. (A friend reports a similar experience with his unused hearing aids, which "so greatly magnified the noise of chewing that I couldn't eat and converse at the same time.")

But my resistance is bound to melt. And surely, having lamented my mother's embarrassed social isolation, I will suffer similar distress. "Not having understood what was said in a group," she reminisces, "I would chime in and say the same thing someone else had just said—and everyone would laugh. I would be so embarrassed, I wanted to fall through the floor." Increasingly, her way of coping was to avoid getting out onto the floor in the first place. She shied away from public events more and more and found excuses not to mix with people who didn't understand, or, when she did go out, would signal my amiable father to take her home while the evening was still young.

Will I do the same? Will I break my private vow not to repeat her past?

In the world of the hearing-impaired, those who have been deaf since birth are my distant cousins. I empathize as I read their stories. But I would not trivialize their experience by identifying it with my own. A great divide separates those who are natively deaf or were deafened before they learned to speak and those who are hard of hearing or were deafened later in life. I can hardly imagine the consciousness of those for whom in the beginning there was no word, only silence. I can no more imagine congenital deafness than a nearsighted person can imagine blindness. Unlike people who have been deaf most of their lives, I have known, and still know, the sound of waves splashing, of symphonies playing, of children laughing. Thus, those most akin to me are the millions of fellow travelers anywhere on the slow voyage from sound to silence, from hearing to nonhearing. It is for them, and for those who love and wish to understand them, that I record my journey toward a silent world.

The Beat Goes On 28 JUNE 1991

My twenty-one-year-old son Andy returns home from a weeklong visit with Seattle relatives. While chauffeuring his grandmother, he discovered a positive side to her deafness—he could play any music as loud as he wished. I chuckle at the image of my ultra-conservative eighty-one-year-old mother riding around Seattle with Led Zeppelin blaring from the car stereo. Then I reflect: Will he—or his child—someday drive me around to the beat of heavy-metal bands? Please, my child, make it Vivaldi.

Remembering how my extended family had already welcomed my older son, Peter, on his successful move to Seattle, I ask: "Did they try to cajole you into moving there?"

"Some of them did," I think I hear him say.

"Some of them did?" I say.

He gives me a blank look.

"Some of them did?" I say again, hoping to confirm my understanding and to draw him out.

Without ever answering, he and his mother exchange smirks. "I know what we need to get Dad for Christmas," he says, "one of those magic-slate writing boards, like the one grandmother has."

Flushed with embarrassment and irritation, I drop the question.

Anxiety and Triumph 27 AUGUST 1991

I have just returned from the American Psychological Association convention, where I delivered an invited lecture in a two-hour prime-time block. As I concluded, I dreaded the twenty-five-minute question-and-answer period with the large and responsive audience. Because the session was taped, I also had to repeat each question into the microphone—a can't-fool-'em hearing test.

Bless my colleagues. Mature, confident people all, their booming voices carried to the front. With few problems, I heard and replied to all their questions.

But today, the first day of class after a year-and-a-half leave from teaching, proves distressing. I enter the classroom wondering whether I will notice any hearing decline since my last semester of teaching. Before asking the thirty-five students in my first class to say their names, I disclose my impairment and ask them to make themselves heard by the people in the back row. That way, they'll hear, and I'll hear, too.

In spite of my request, the diffident first student says her name softly. I apologize and ask her to repeat it. The next name I hear, but the following one I miss. One for three. Progressing through the other thirty-odd students, I bat no better than 50 percent. As my distress increases—my body tensing, perspiring—I find myself occasionally pretending that I hear, while desperately searching the class list for a name that sounds like the one I think I heard. I'm most assuredly not learning anyone's name. Nor do I need to, for I also take photos of the students and have them sign a sheet according to where they sat that day.

The next hour I meet with a different group of students. What relief! This time, the first student does exactly as I request—turns and speaks clearly to the person farthest across the room. The second and third students emulate her example. I hear!

Another Way of Teaching? 5 SEPTEMBER 1991

Alas, during the several ensuing class sessions I sometimes discern students' comments, sometimes not. If it is imperative for me to hear and respond, I seek clarification. If I take the unheard comment to be intended for the whole class, I smile and nod, on the assumption that the speaker and the class have already benefited from the remark, even if I haven't. Why embarrass myself and take up their time by having the statement repeated just for me, when perhaps I still wouldn't hear it?

More and more I find myself dreading class. I compare the stress of it, and the distraction of preparing for it, to the pleasure and significance of teaching through my textbooks for introductory and social psychology, whose success has been gratifying.

Keeping up with the whole field of psychology for new editions every three years is nearly a full-time job, I tell myself. Why not make it full-time? What could be more fulfilling than helping teach this personally relevant discipline to several hundred thousand students a year? How many teachers are afforded a more stimulating challenge and meaningful responsibility? Leaving behind the stresses of classroom instruction would be not a retreat from teaching, but an affirmation of my teaching through writing. Who could ask for a more satisfying mission or avenue for creativity? How fortunate I am—I don't *need* to do my teaching live in a classroom, for I am blessed with a calling and a means of support that fuel my work outside the classroom.

Or so I indulge myself in thinking after a stressful day in class. But no, insists Carol. It's important for your students—and for your writing—that you stay connected with people who represent the unseen ones you write for. It's also important for your family relationships, she remarks for the 273rd time, that you explore the new hearing technology.

Connection — 5 SEPTEMBER 1991 (Later)

"Only connect!" begins Henry Kisor's memoir of deafness (quoting E. M. Forster). "Only connect, and the beast and the monk, robbed of the isolation that is life to either, will die." I cannot deny it. Several years ago I wrote, with Martin Bolt, a little book of social-psychological essays titled *The Human Connection.*

So, today, I yield to the pleas and nagging of my family. I call the local ear, nose, and throat office and request, as Carol's internist has suggested, a referral to a "tertiary center." The receptionist can't imagine what I'm talking about. I explain—a place that evaluates patients and specializes in outfitting people with the latest in hearing technology.

"How does that differ from what we do?" she asks. I feel as if I've just called a nearby restaurant and asked the hostess to refer me to a place to eat—a place that serves *good* food. The medical receptionist kindly says she'll check with the audiologist and call me back.

Waiting 5 NOVEMBER 1991

For nearly two months I hear nothing back. At least, though, I have my family off my back. After I made *the* call, the ball was in someone else's court. Until a couple days ago—when the audiologist finally returned my call and invited me to go in for a hearing evaluation.

Today's testing reveals (in comparison with previous test records dating back twenty-five years) a further deterioration in the hearing in my left ear, but little change in the right ear. I hadn't realized that I have, relatively speaking, a bad ear and a better ear. Carol has been wanting me to explore the new programmable aids ever since reading about Ronald Reagan's. The audiologist, who concurs that I am a candidate for one, refers me to a Grand Rapids clinic. There, the next day I experience another round of testing and am fitted for an $1,100 instrument for my left ear.

Selective Amplification 21 NOVEMBER 1991

I return to Grand Rapids to receive the aid, which the audiologist programs. This, I'm told, is one of only 9,000 in-the-ear programmable aids in the nation.

A computer, through wires attached to the aid, first generates and records sounds, automatically adjusting the aid's output in response to my ear's acoustical structure. I am given a hearing test recording my hearing threshold for each of thirteen frequencies. Finally, a check is performed to minimize feedback (the whistle sound that hearing aids sometimes make when covered). Then, at the touch of a button, the computer program is transferred to the microchip in my ear. The microphone goes on, amplifying sound selectively (rather like the graphic equalizer in a stereo) in response to my hearing loss at each frequency.

Driving home, I find the "roar" of the car and the wind distracting. If this be hearing, give me silence! Even more distracting is the sound of my own voice. It's like talking with your head in a bucket. Or like having a bad sinus cold, which amplifies the resonance of your own voice. (Don't be shocked at this, say books on hearing loss: if things sound "unnatural" with a hearing aid, it's by comparison with the now impaired definition of "natural.")

On the positive side, I must admit that I also hear better things I *want* to hear better. I turn down the car radio. At home, I hear the television at a lower volume—a fact that, by itself, would justify the $1,100 as far as Carol is concerned. (I also sometimes use a remote-hearing device that, by receiving an infrared signal from the television, allows me to dial my own volume, independent of the volume on the set.)

Adjustment and the "Earlid" Effect 24 NOVEMBER 1991

I return for a follow-up appointment with the audiologist. After a week of using the hearing aid, I acknowledge that I can hear better, but lament the amplification of my own voice. Is that something I will adapt to, much as I've adapted to a new glasses prescription? Yes, it takes time, he says.

And once I have adapted, might I then use the instrument selectively? When we were living in Scotland, it took months for driving on the left-hand side to become automatic. After it did, I feared that back in the United States I would have to readjust to driving on the right. But no—I retained my "schema" for driving on the right and had no problem, except for occasionally starting to get in on the wrong side of the car. When we revisit Scotland, I am still comfortable driving on the left.

Might I similarly become comfortable both with and without the aid in my ear? I could use it when connecting—when teaching, in meetings, at home—and I could *not* use it when I was working in my office and wanted to shut out distracting noises. God saw fit to give us eyelids to shut out unwanted light but not earlids to banish unwanted sound. Are hearing-aided people, who can turn sound up or down, enjoying the closest approximation to earlids? (The Scottish biblical scholar-writer William Barclay noted, in *Daily Readings with William Barclay* (1973), the benefits of not hearing: "I am almost completely deaf. But this means I can sleep without trouble in a noisy hotel by a railway station! And I can concentrate far better on work and study for I have no distractions. . . . A handicap has its compensations.")

Yes, you could try using the aid selectively, like an earlid, says the audiologist.

Hits, Misses, and Spousal Involvement — 28 NOVEMBER 1991

After Thanksgiving dinner I mention to Carol that I think I hardly hear better with the aid—I miss as much as before. The arrival of the aid has hardly meant "here today, hear tomorrow." I am reminded of the man who expounded to a friend on the wonders of his new electronic hearing device. "That's wonderful!" replied the friend. "What kind is it?" Looking at his watch, the man said, "It's ten past two."

Carol responds as the audiologist did: What you haven't previously heard you don't count as a "miss." (It's hard to notice the dog's *not* barking—the clue that enabled Sherlock Holmes, the only person who noticed, to solve the Silver Blaze case.) The spouse who says something and gets no response records a miss. The nonhearing person does not—but scores as "hits" things that are heard. Thus, the perceived hit-to-miss ratio is deceptively high for the hard of hearing.

As part of their marketing strategy, hearing-aid companies therefore insist on involving the spouse. Spouses are more aware of what's missed, more receptive to the sales pitch, and more likely to seal the deal. When talking with married hearing-aid wearers, I've often said, "Let me guess: your wife/husband got you to do this." Inevitably, the reply is a sheepish nod.

Failing to hear what your partner hears helps drive the point home. The difficulty of detecting your own hearing loss is like the difficulty of noticing slight deterioration in visual acuity. Playing alphabet game in the car, I am astonished that others can read billboards a hundred yards before I can read them. In the absence of such comparisons, my vision seems normal—isn't this how other people see?

The understandable failure to notice hearing "misses" helps explain the "denial" often attributed to the hearing-impaired. "If you refuse to admit that you cannot hear well and persist in blaming other people for not speaking clearly or loudly enough, you are in a psychological state known as denial," states Marcia Dugan in her helpful book, *Keys to Living with Hearing Loss.* Well, yes, but one needn't, à la Freud, attribute denial to repression of a painful reality. Denial may instead be rooted in ignorance of how many things go unheard.

Here, in Carol's own words, is the spousal strategy she used to help puncture my not-so-blissful ignorance:

> David, not unlike other people experiencing increasing hearing loss, resisted having his hearing tested, acknowledging his need for hearing assistance, and taking steps to get hearing aids. As his loss progressed, David was missing more and more and needing to have many more things repeated. I was embarrassed for him as he would respond inappropriately or begin talking about another topic while everyone else was having a conversation.
>
> Most of our friends were aware of his loss, so they understood what was going on. Increasingly, though, I was hearing comments that David was missing more. Simply telling him that he really should get a hearing aid was not effective. Increased nagging about it wouldn't have helped, either, and would have injected an ongoing negative tenor into our lives. So I made the decision to tell David each time he misheard something or missed it altogether. No more was I going to just cover, or repeat or explain what had happened. Instead, I would calmly say, "David, you didn't hear what Andy said. He said . . ." Or, when we could come home, I'd report, "When you said . . . , what had really been asked was . . ." It was my version of "tough love." I had decided that the most productive, caring response was to try to help force David out of denial about the extent of his hearing loss and help him confront this reality so that he would be willing to take positive steps to address his needs. It worked.

Facing Reality 7 JANUARY 1992

The first day of a new term forces me to meet one class of thirty-three students, for which I self-consciously wear the aid. Although I have by now adapted to it around the house, where I faithfully wear it with diminishing awareness of my own distorted voice, the stress and self-consciousness induced by the evaluative audience—the students sizing me up on the first day of class—again makes me aware of the head-in-the-bucket effect. Distracted, I notice myself stammering through a number of grammatically incorrect sentences in a less than sterling performance. Afterward, I ask my assistant if I talk differently—too loud? too soft? She assures me that she can't tell the difference.

Fortunately, the second class has but sixteen students, which I group in a tight circle around me. Aided by a class list, I dispense with the aid and join them in a name-learning exercise. Alas, to hear who they are, I still have to have some of them repeat their names. One student, not on the list, introduces himself as "Leo," but when I use that name, he corrects me and says it again. Thinking that I've said someone else's name, I rectify, Ah, yes, Leo. Not until I misuse it again does someone get through to me that it's Theo. Another male student, immediately to my right, contributes to the discussion in such a soft, low voice that I barely get the gist of his remarks. Although the lecture part of the class goes better—I feel strong and articulate—I realize that, even in this small class, I'm going to have to endure the device.

Speaking to forty adults in a church class, I struggle again. My distress rising after three repetitions of a question from the back, I sheepishly ask someone in the front to repeat the question. Definitely a bad hear day.

Confrontation 9 JANUARY 1992

I must have forgotten to turn off the radio in leaving the car—something I always try to remember, so that Carol doesn't get blasted out when she's the next person to use the car. In bed last night she lights into me, first concerning the decibel level. She's read an article about how sound over 85 decibels can damage the cochlea's hair receptors—true, though I explain to her that I play the radio at a fraction of that or for that matter of the Amy Grant concert I took our daughter Laura to last fall (even I found that almost painfully deafening). This was an interesting reversal of an opposite theory that she offered earlier (based on a friend's report of a conversation with a hearing-aid specialist)—namely, that hearing aids, by amplifying sound, help keep the ear's receptors from atrophying. When I told that one to my audiologist, he disputed it, as I expected, and quipped, "That sounds like someone trying to sell hearing aids." (Prolonged and profound sound deprivation does, however, reduce the brain's ability to process sound.)

Her other expressed concern is with safety: "With the radio that loud, I know I couldn't hear a siren or a horn. I'm concerned that you might have an accident." Defensively, I insist that I can hear a siren or horn perfectly well—I can even hear the tires meeting the road. Moreover, I have good vision. I drive carefully. And in recent years I have had a perfect driving record. Besides, is she suggesting that members of the deaf community (which I have not yet joined) should be banned from driving? "How about a little more empathy and a little less judgment," I grumpily suggest. "Don't you want me to be concerned with your safety?" she rejoins.

Well, I tell her, if she thinks my hearing is so bad as that, then she should have some understanding of why I am enjoying classroom teaching less and less and why I might want to shift away from teaching conversationally (in classrooms) to teaching predominantly through my writing. My teaching seems to be beginning a downhill slide. Although formal student evaluations of my teaching last semester were still gratifying, they were down a bit from previous student evaluations. Meanwhile, my writing still seems to be going well. As one who feels called to teach this humanly significant discipline through my texts, should I not concentrate most of my energies on them? That is the direction in which I am led.

Or is Carol right that I still have something important to offer students face to face? (I'm less sure of my irreplaceability, especially given the competence of some of my department colleagues). If she is right that it's important for me as a writer to stay in touch with students, are there not other ways to do so (through all the feedback I receive from other campuses, for example)? Maybe my being here at Hope College and talking with students daily is as effective a way of staying attuned to students' concerns as teaching in the classroom.

Good News, Bad News 22 JANUARY 1992

The good news: I'm increasingly readapting to the sound of my own voice. In class, I'm less and less distracted, and better able to hear. At the adult class at our church, where I've decided to endure the head-in-the-bucket effect to minimize the risk of again not hearing, the slight decline in articulateness is more than offset by my ability to participate more effectively in dialogue.

The bad news: with or without the hearing aid, I obviously don't hear as other people do. Night before last, I attended, with several hundred others, a Martin Luther King, Jr., anniversary service in our college chapel. The singing of a large gospel choir was terrific, though I could hardly make out a word. The speaker seemed well received, but when you miss 40 percent of the words—even with the hearing aid—the mind continually wanders. Even when struggling to hear, I couldn't make out what it was I was supposed to say. But everyone else heard. So when the speaker asked us to stand and say something to the people around us, I offered lamely, and inappropriately, "I'm Dave," whereas they all said (I was later told), "Activate your faith." At home afterward, Carol argued that there *is* a point to continuing to attend such public events, not only to offer a supportive witness, but also to share in community worship, as Mother has done even throughout her years of utter deafness. Still, remembering how off-key her singing became as she lost her ear for music, I sing softly.

The "Disability" Label 26 MARCH 1992

As I wear "it" more and more—to church education classes and fellowship groups, to talks I attend or give—the self-consciousness-inducing head-in-the-bucket effect is lessening. I am adapting.

I am also, however, experiencing a phenomenon that the audiologist predicted (and of which I'm glad he forewarned me). Although I still miss many things with the aid, I feel as though I'm missing more than ever without it. I have the sense that my hearing decline is accelerating, as if the aid were wearing out my ear. "Once they adapt to an aid, people often think their hearing without the aid has gotten much worse—when tests show it hasn't," I recall the audiologist's saying.

Yesterday, after I showed my classes a video of courageous disabled people (three of Britain's limbless Thalidomide children now living happy, productive adult lives), we discussed humanity's enormous capacity to adapt to changed circumstances. After a year of adaptation to their new life, people who have won a state lottery or been paralyzed in an auto accident hardly differ from other people in their capacity for joy. It's astonishing, and something we can all take comfort in, given our vulnerability to tragedy or disability. I take consolation from that reality, I tell the class, because I believe that I am in the early stages of going deaf, and that my family and social relationships will be impeded, my teaching career cut short.

Janet's hand shoots up, and she recalls having had a high school teacher who was deaf. "But how could she teach?" I ask. By reading lips, and notes on slips of paper, Janet explains. What courage, I say, though I'm inclined to think that by the time I reached that point, my students would be better served by whoever would replace me.

Carol later wonders whether, when that happens, I will take disability pay. Disability? The idea of eventually drawing disability has never occurred to me, nor have I thought of myself as becoming "disabled." When the Americans with Disabilities Act came into effect this spring, I thought, "How nice for those people in wheelchairs and those with Seeing Eye dogs."

2
Relationships

Rooted in Relationships 6 MAY 1992

Life is getting easier, and harder. Easier, as book royalties bring in much more money than we have any need for. I remain a person of reasonably simple pleasures: I care little for clothes or cars. If a fire destroyed such possessions, my self would be intact. But take away my family, my closest friends, my work, my faith, and you *would* destroy my sense of self. For it is in my human connections—through my close relationships and my writing and teaching—and in my spiritual connection with God that I know who and why I am. Still, it's nice to have no financial needs or worries.

Yet life is getting a little harder, too. Although I felt gratified by student ratings at the end of the semester just completed, teaching is more of a struggle, and I engage the students in dialogue less than I used to. At a recent dinner party, surrounded by the buzz of conversation, I had difficulty making out the words of my hostess, though she was speaking into my aided ear from about a foot away.

Jokingly referring to a heavily advertised hearing aid, I later tell Carol I need a "Miracle Ear clarifier" that will screen out all the conversations but the one I'm listening to. And I wonder again: Will I, like Mother, come to avoid such social occasions and force my spouse to take me home early? Will my sense of self become less rooted in relationships? Perhaps. Already, I understand Mother better.

Book Tour 27 MAY 1992

I have just returned from a short publicity tour for my book *The Pursuit of Happiness.* Despite my anxieties (and my wondering still whether all that money and time could have been better devoted to other ways of promoting the book), the tour seemed to go well. On radio talk shows, all the stations I visited enabled the guest to control the volume on the headset. Only once, when doing a radio interview from my hotel room, was I flustered at being almost unable to hear the interviewer. (I must learn to forewarn interviewers of my need for volume and clarity.) That was enough to make me think that this first publicity tour was in all likelihood my last.

Now, this evening, I am due to be on an interview with call-ins on the 5:30 news and feature segment of our local NBC affiliate. My fear is that with no headset and no way to control volume, I may miss what some of the callers say. If so, it will disrupt the show's rapid-fire format, deprive me of speaking time, and generally embarrass us all.

Afterward: For the first time, a live (six-minute) interview does not go well (wouldn't you know it—the only one my family and friends would hear). The questions (from listeners troubled by their alcoholism, bereavement, and friends' depression) went beyond my topic and my expertise, my answers were off the mark, and the setup—with an ear bug for the calls, which fed my own voice back to me—was distracting. Worse, Carol was surprised that I had nothing helpful to say to the woman who wanted to know how to help her depressed friend. "Was that what she asked?" I groaned, realizing that I had responded inappropriately on-air.

A Candle Extinguished 26 JUNE 1992

One of my distant hopes has been that cochlear-implant technology, now in its infancy, may someday develop to the point where it would benefit people like me as we complete the transition to deafness. (A cochlear implant transmits signals from a sound-processing unit to a coil attached to the skull. From this external coil an electrode reaches into the malfunctioning inner ear, where it stimulates the auditory nerve.) Happily, one of the leading researcher-practitioners of cochlear implants for the profoundly deaf has been John Kemink, a University of Michigan physician who is a Hope College graduate and supporter and also young enough that he may still be around when I need him. Last fall, when I was considering what sort of new aid to consider, I sent Kemink my hearing profiles, dating back twenty-five years. He replied, recommending the programmable aid. It was good to know that someone within the greater Hope College community was at the forefront of treatment for the profoundly deaf.

Was until yesterday, when he was murdered—shot three times—in his Michigan Medical Center office (by a patient who was upset by Kemink's having referred him to another physician who had failed to cure the man's problem). Although my sense of loss is nominal compared with that of his wife and two young children, I did feel it in my stomach as I saw the headline in this morning's *Detroit Free Press.* A freakish event, stealing the life of the one brilliant doctor who, of all physicians, just happened to be my secret hope for the future.

Trying to Understand 30 JUNE 1992

I was on back-to-back hour-long radio talk shows last week. I was talking from my office with interviewers and listeners in Urbana, Illinois, and in Pittsburgh, Pennsylvania. Well, *trying* to talk. The first went tolerably well, but the second gave me a headache. Even with my phone volume turned up high, I could not hear—or at best, could barely hear—the callers. I struggled to grasp their questions, to know when they had stopped talking and were waiting for a response, and to know when they were talking to the interviewer rather than to me. For some, the problem was mutual—they couldn't hear me.

Would hearing people have had equal difficulty on a normal phone? Am I attributing the failed communication to my poor hearing, rather than to the station's poor equipment? How much should I worry about pending talk shows? The hard of hearing can err in either direction—by denying their disability or by blaming too much on it.

Interpreting Responses 11 JULY 1992

Further musings about the ambiguities of interpreting people's responses to hearing impairment. Yesterday I was following the flow nicely in a talk show interview on a large St. Louis station. The hosts and the first two callers projected well. As the third caller offered her prescription for happy living, I turned my phone volume control up to 10 and switched the phone from the familiar left-ear position to what I now realize is my better (right) ear. (Anyone who thinks it's easy to concentrate while talking on the phone with the "wrong ear" should try it.) Unfortunately, I didn't catch what she said. As I dreaded, one of the hosts then solicited my opinion: "What about that, Dr. Myers?" When I confessed that I couldn't hear, the host repeated some platitudes. I concurred with them—whereupon, eight minutes before the hour was up, the host abruptly thanked me for being with them and ended the interview.

Yet another response to my impaired hearing? Or am I being paranoid—maybe they actually had other commentary and ads to squeeze in before the top of the hour?

My mind drifts to two provocative experiments. In the first, Dartmouth College researchers Robert Kleck and Angelo Strenta led college women to feel disfigured. The women thought that the purpose of the experiment was to assess how other people react to a severe facial scar created with theatrical makeup. Actually, the purpose was to see how the women themselves, when made to feel abnormal, perceived others' behavior toward them. After applying the makeup, the experimenter gave each subject a small hand mirror so that she could see the realistic-looking scar. Once she put the mirror down, he applied some "moisturizer to keep the makeup from cracking." What the "moisturizer" really did was remove the scar.

The scenes that followed were poignant. A young woman, feeling terribly self-conscious about her supposedly disfigured face, would be talking with another woman, who saw no such disfigurement and knew nothing of what had gone on before. All of us who have ever felt similarly self-conscious, perhaps over acne or "awful-looking" hair—or a disability such as a hearing impairment—can sympathize. Compared with women who were led to believe that their conversational partners merely thought they had an allergy, the "disfigured" women became acutely sensitive to how their partners were looking at them. They rated their conversational partners as tenser, more distant, and more patronizing than did the control group. But in fact, observers who later analyzed videotapes of the interactions with "disfigured" persons could observe no such differences in treatment. Hyperaware of being different from other people, the "disfigured" women overreacted to mannerisms and comments that they would otherwise not have noticed. Sometimes we perceive others as reacting to our distinctiveness when they actually aren't.

In the second experiment, reported in *Science* (1981), Philip Zimbardo, a creative social psychologist, wondered about the finding that paranoid reactions commonly accompany gradual hearing loss later in life. Is the paranoia a natural response to not hearing what people are saying in your presence? To find out, Zimbardo used hypnotic suggestion to induce an experience of partial deafness in eighteen highly hypnotizable male Stanford University students. If unaware what was causing their hearing difficulty, the men became more suspicious of others' apparently hushed voices and consequently more irritable and unfriendly. Men who were made aware of the source of their hearing difficulty, by contrast, did not show such paranoia. It is those whose hearing is declining but who do not yet want to admit it who are most likely to begin feeling suspicious and irritable, it seems. In real life, it often takes a gentle, loving, honest friend to alert them to the change they are undergoing.

Howard Hughes' withdrawal and paranoia appear to have been partly attributable to a hearing impairment. In a letter published by *Hearing Health,* his onetime friend Katharine Hepburn reports that Hughes began losing his hearing at about age fifteen. "When I knew him just before he was 30, he was noticeably deaf. He was embarrassed by it and seemed to find asking people to speak up an agony. As time went on, he retreated to the telephone on which he could turn up the sound. By this unfortunate retreat, he became lonely and finally remote from the actualities of normal life." If only he had responded as had his uncle Rupert Hughes, who had introduced him to the motion picture business. Rupert had also suffered hearing loss, but he took to wearing a cumbersome hearing aid. When he died in 1956, he had "more friends than anyone in Hollywood."

Clarification Wanted 21 JULY 1992

Another radio talk show, "with Chuck so-and-so. . . . Chuck, rhymes with Jed," explains the producer in Rochester, New York, and with a woman whose name I don't get. Ah, but when I'm patched into the on-air dialogue, I hear her clearly identify herself as Carol so-and-so. After I mention her name in on-air conversation, Chuck—whose named turns out to be Chet (rhymes with jet)—comes on during the first break to tell me that he enjoyed reading my book—and that his partner's name is not Carol but Tara.

I apologize and later reflect that even if I someday write another book for general readers, I will not submit—with hearing that has deteriorated still further—to another round of talk shows. The problem, as many a hearing-impaired person will confirm, is not so much an inability to *hear* sound as an inability to carve meaning out of sound. (The ease and speed with which the hearing brain parses and decodes the vocal sound stream is one of the world's great wonders.) Talking with Chet, Tara, and their callers, I had plenty of volume in my ear, thanks to a strong signal from the station and the volume control on my phone. I wouldn't have wanted their voices any louder. Still, even strong sounds sometimes seem muffled. No wonder there seems to be such a market these days for that hearing aid cleverly hyped as the "Miracle Ear clarifier." Note—not a "magnifier" (because the hard of hearing don't want just more intense sound)—but a device that promises to ungarble, to unscramble, to clarify human vocal sounds.

Catching the Meaning 8 AUGUST 1992

While vacationing in Washington, my old home state, I again read Henry Kisor's *What's that Pig Outdoors? A Memoir of Deafness* (1990). Kisor, a Chicago journalist, lost his hearing to meningitis when he was three but became sufficiently skilled at lipreading to succeed in regular classes, right through Northwestern University's graduate school of journalism and into a career as a book editor and a columnist for the *Chicago Sun-Times.* I mark a handful of paragraphs:

> It's far easier for the lipreader to understand someone if he already knows the subject of the conversation, for he can anticipate the words used to discuss it. If the subject is, for example, the Chicago Bears, a deaf pro football enthusiast will consciously be watching for proper names such as "Ditka" or even "Wojciechowski"—words he'd never understand in any other context." (p. xiv)

It's true for the hearing-impaired as well. When we have the right mental set (what psychologists call a schema), we can more easily catch the meaning. To some extent, it's true for anyone. Whether we hear the speaker saying "cults and sects" or "cults and sex" depends on the context. Such contextual cues become more important for listeners who don't hear well.

> Those who favor American Sign Language, which has a syntax of its own utterly unlike English, complain that total communication forces its users to sign in English word order, an almost incomprehensible pidgin version of ASL. (p. 9)

This fact helps explain the difficulty of learning fluent sign language later in life. The early years are critical for mastering the grammar and syntax of any language. In one study, by Jacqueline Johnson and Elissa Newport, Korean and Chinese immigrants to the United States took a grammar test requiring them to identify each of 276 sentences (for example, "Yesterday the hunter shoots a deer") as correct or incorrect. Ten years after immigrating, those who had immigrated and learned English in early childhood showed near-perfect knowledge of correct English grammar. Those who had immigrated as adults, many of whom were professors or mature graduate students, had much greater difficulty.

Likewise, deaf children who learn sign language from birth master the subtle grammar of sign language better than those who learn ASL as teens or adults: just as it is more difficult for adult immigrants to learn and speak a new language than it is for their children, so it is more difficult for those of us who lose our hearing as adults to become fluent in sign language. I'm too busy now to take time to learn signing. Yet if Carol and I want to learn it at all—and she's the one I would lean on for interpretation—we'd best not wait until, like Mother, I find hearing aids useless. By then, we'll be reduced to magic slates (or, I trust, some newer, more efficient keyboard and display device).

> Blindness is a handicap of mobility, deafness one of communication. . . . In the hearing world, deaf people tend to be solitary and ignored if they are lucky, lonely and rejected if they are not. That is why Samuel Johnson called deafness "the most desperate of human calamities." (pp. 10–11)

> Those who hear cannot imagine how grindingly lonely deafness often can be. . . . Just as do the hearing, the deaf

> need to communicate, to share their thoughts and feelings with others. Only a fellow lifer in the jailhouse of silence understands how important that is to sanity and how difficult it can be to achieve. (pp. 152–53)

I have only tasted this experience, but enough to have the feeling of marginality when, with or without a hearing device, a group's conversation is beyond the reach of my ears. At such times, hating to interrupt constantly for clarification, one sits back and, feeling a little sad and lonely, watches the others enjoying themselves.

> [My worried future in-laws] would have been even more concerned had they known that the divorce rate of deaf-and-hearing marriages is close to 90 percent. Such marriages tend to break down for the usual reasons: because of a lack of understanding, communication, and flexibility between the partners. (p. 157)

Although Carol and I both come from hearing cultures, I can believe that communication problems strain the marriages of the deaf—and of the hearing-impaired. I believe it from having experienced minor communication breakdowns in our own marriage, and from observing the reduced communication between my faithful father and my mother. Although I can't say how *I* would react if I were the spouse with acute hearing, I do empathize with Dad and Carol and all spouses of the hearing-impaired. Loneliness and frustration curse not just the deaf.

Maintaining an Optimistic Outlook 13 AUGUST 1992

The plague is obviously genetic. On that visit to Seattle and Bainbridge Island last week, I took (as requested) pamphlets describing my programmable aid to my sister and a brother. My sister, Nancy, a fifty-seven-year-old with the bounce and vitality of a forty-year-old, has an aid that she seldom wears. Brother Dick, fifty-five, is curious—but his wife, Jan, is clearly more than curious. Like Carol, she is eager, hoping that I can convert my brother. In an attempt to do my part, I wear my aid at nearly all times in their presence.

One volume of *Genetics of Hearing Impairment* reports this from a national survey of children in schools for the deaf: the odds of two deaf parents having a deaf child are one in ten. The odds rise to six in ten for the next child of those whose first child is born deaf. A British study yielded similar estimates. For any given couple, these odds will vary, depending on the cause of their deafness. Although I am unaware of any similarly precise estimates for the hard of hearing, our family's experience—which I have entered into the government-financed Boys Town Research Registry for Hereditary Hearing Loss—suggests the hereditary pattern that many other families have noticed.

A third sibling, Jim, forty-five, seems untroubled by hearing loss. Instead, a worse scourge has struck, one that may render irrelevant the possibility of deafness later in life. Jim suffers from one of nature's horrible afflictions, motor neuron disease. For most people, the disease progressively erodes the capacity to control the limbs and, in the end, even to speak or breathe—all the while leaving their senses and minds fully alert to their own degeneration. Its best-known form is amyotrophic lateral sclerosis (ALS)—Lou Gehrig's disease.

Now in an early stage of the disease, Jim has difficulty

tying his shoes, buttoning his shirt, and typing in his job as promotions director at a network television station. Nevertheless, what continually amazes me is the resilience of his spirit, the joy he takes in being with his young daughters, the enthusiasm he feels for his volunteer church work, the happiness he finds in knowing that his initial prognosis was too grim and that a new experimental drug may be slowing the course of his disease and giving him the great gift of seeing his daughters grow to maturity. After staring death in the face, he knows what matters. "Life itself seems more precious and real," he says. As fellow motor neuron disease survivor Stephen Hawking put it, "When one's expectations are reduced to zero, one really appreciates everything that one does have."

By comparison, my problem is trivial, and my hopes for future joy are therefore perhaps greater. If sufferers from motor neuron disease can achieve a perspective that sustains peace and joy, surely I can, too. I believe this, even though I acknowledge my frustration at missing the punch line in a joke that everyone else is guffawing over or feel embarrassed after making what I later learn is an inappropriate reply to a soft-spoken person whose words I thought I had heard.

Perseverance Produces Payoffs 22 AUGUST 1992

This morning I had a new experience. (In time, I suppose my entries will become less frequent, as I have progressively fewer first times.) Here at a retreat center in the Berkshire Hills of eastern New York, I am participating in the annual Worth Publishers sales meeting. At breakfast, shortly before a four-hour discussion of the marketing of my introductory psychology text, my hearing-aid battery went dead. Fortunately, I had a spare. But it, too, was dead! A mild panic swept over me: "I won't be able to hear many of the questions and comments."

Happily, a nearby drugstore was open early, enabling me to put my aid back in business. How ironic, I reflected, driving back from the store, that today I felt as though I couldn't cope without an instrument that less than a year ago I felt as though I couldn't cope *with.* Perhaps there is a lesson here for anyone adapting to new hearing aids, new glasses, new anything. Hang in there. Persist—it will get better.

A Frustrating Experience 24 SEPTEMBER 1992

Last night Carol and I heard (well, she did) our distinguished college organist, Huw Lewis, give an explanation of the history and technology of organs, punctuated by demonstrations on the college's main organ. Our cavernous Gothic chapel provides wonderful depth for music, but not for speech. As Lewis's voice boomed over the public address system, at more than adequate volume, then echoed off the walls, I was able to grasp words only in clumps, with or without my aid. Obviously others around me could hear, for they were laughing at his jokes, none of which I caught. When he explained the attributes of a type of pipe, then turned to play that pipe, I hadn't a clue what he was demonstrating.

The evening was for me largely a frustrating waste. At

such times, I sometimes occupy my mind by wondering, How could these other people possibly extract meaning from that echoing sound? Although today's state-of-the-art hearing technology does its best to simulate normal hearing, it still falls short. Will the technology of 2010 do better?

Hope 7 NOVEMBER 1992

Hope springs eternal. A new report in *Science* reveals that in some animals, such as young chickens, the sensory cells of the inner ear can regenerate themselves. This finding raises hopes that sensorineural ("nerve deafness") hearing loss might someday be curable. Armed with this knowledge, researchers are searching for the chemical signals that rouse the inner ear from its dormant state to begin producing new hair cells. No one has yet induced this regeneration in mammals, so the human ear may be incapable of renewing itself. Still, the researchers' dream is to discover a way to trick mammalian ears into doing what chick's ears can do, thereby making improved hearing possible for those of us with sensorineural loss. Stay tuned.

P.S. (13 January 1999) Writing in *The Consumer Handbook on Hearing Loss and Hearing Aids* (1998), University of Washington researcher Edwin Rubel reports that there are now twenty to thirty research teams, including his own, exploring possible hair-cell regeneration in mammalian cochlea. He guesses "that within 5 to 10 years, we'll find out if it's possible to regenerate hair cells at [levels] sufficient to restore hearing in mammals. From there, it could be as little as another 10 years until we achieve hair cell regeneration in humans. If successful, it could eliminate some of the need for hearing aids and cochlear implants as we now know them."

Stem-cell research also suggests the possibility of signaling mammalian cells to differentiate into hair cells that could be placed in the inner ear. There they might signal existing nerve fibers to transmit information to the brain. Another possibility envisaged is the transplanting of embryonic mammalian hair cells into the adult ear.

Debates on Attitude and Terminology 9 NOVEMBER 1992

More on cochlear implants. Last night's *60 Minutes* program featured a seven-year-old girl who completely lost her hearing in infancy (as did Henry Kisor) when she contracted meningitis. Thanks to a cochlear implant, her hearing has been partially restored, and, after training, her capacity to understand speech (even over the phone with no visual cues) is remarkable. Knowing the comparatively greater "plasticity" of children's brains and the resultant capacity for learning, however, I will be surprised if deaf senior citizens derive similar benefits from today's cochlear implants.

Objecting to the operation, deaf culture spokespersons associated with the National Association of the Deaf argued that deafness is not a disability. It could as well be considered "vision enhancement" as "hearing impairment." In an essay in *Genetics of Hearing Impairment,*

Gallaudet University president I. King Jordan recalls an earlier *60 Minutes* interview with Meredith Vieira:

> She asked me this question: "If there [were] a pill that you could take and you would wake up with normal hearing, would you take it?" I told her that her question upset me. I told her that it was something I spent virtually no time at all thinking about, and I asked her if she would ask me the same question about a "white" pill if I were a black man. Then I asked if, as a woman, she would take a "man" pill. Our conversation continued long after the videotaping was done, and we have had several subsequent conversations. But she never understood. She still does not. She still thinks only from her own frame of reference and imagines that not hearing would be a terrible thing. Deafness is not simply the opposite of hearing. It is much more than that, and those of us who live and work and play and lead full lives as deaf people try very hard to communicate this fact.

Well, of course, I reflect. She doesn't fathom his experience. But does *he* grasp her experience of hearing? If he did, would he still feel no wish to hear?

At least this much can be said: there is a growing consensus that native signers are not linguistically disabled. "It is quite natural," wrote Gertrude Stein. "Some hear more pleasantly with the eyes than with the ears." Gallaudet College linguist William Stokoe confirmed the naturalness of visual language in his groundbreaking book *Sign Language Structure* (1960), which showed that Sign is a complete language with its own grammar, syntax, and semantics.

A year ago I sent my text coverage of deafness to one of the *60 Minutes* interviewees, Harlan Lane. He replied graciously, but questioned my presenting deaf people as "hearing-impaired." To people at the core of the deaf culture, "the term 'hearing-impaired' is offensive," he said. "Blacks are not 'white-impaired,' they argue, nor women 'male-impaired.'" When I passed these thoughts along to John Kemink shortly before his murder, he noted that "having a different ethnic, racial, or cultural background is a different situation from being deaf (a loss of one of the five senses)."

Yes, there are similarities, but "also real differences." And why, I wondered later, don't blind people similarly celebrate blindness, by insisting that blindness is not visual impairment but hearing enhancement?[1] As some deaf parents rejoice when their child is born deaf, why don't blind parents feel glad when their child is born blind? (When those who are blind or in wheelchairs are asked if they wish they could see or walk, they usually unhesitatingly answer Yes.)

Part of me is pleased to hear further testimony to something I mentioned earlier—the remarkable human ability to adapt to new circumstances. And there is some evidence from studies of "compensation" (reported in the September 1992 issue of *Psychological Bulletin*) that people for whom one channel of sensation is closed off will partly compensate through a slight enhancement of their other sensory abilities. The parts of Helen Keller's brain

1. In *Touching the Rock* (Vintage Books, 1990), John Hull reports after six years of living with blindness that "if blindness is a gift, it is not one that I would wish on anybody. It is not a gift I want to receive. It is something which I would rather like to give back, but one which I find I cannot help accepting." Later, however, he did come to see some partial compensations. "Increasingly, I do not think of myself so much as a blind person, which would define me with reference to sighted people and as lacking something, but simply as a whole-body-seer. . . . Blindness is the wrapping, or the medium. The gift lies deeper, on the other side of blindness."

that were not receiving visual and auditory input were available for other uses, such as discriminating between touch sensations. Perhaps visual compensation explains why there are so many visually skilled deaf engineers, deaf architects, and deaf mathematicians. New research at the University of Montreal indicates that, with one ear plugged, blind people are more accurate than sighted people at locating a sound source.

By comparison with blind people, however, people who are deaf from birth seem to exhibit fewer compensatory sensory enhancements. For example, they apparently don't exhibit superior reading ability (which is nurtured as people learn the spoken language). Moreover, unlike those who are congenitally deaf, people who have had and lost their hearing would surely admit to having a disability. Who among them would not welcome an artificial ear that, like an artificial heart, could replace their malfunctioning organ? Such people, not having learned fluent signing from an early age, surely *are* handicapped by deafness. They needn't think of themselves as disabled *people* to acknowledge that they have a disability (a description of the impairment, not the person). This reasoning explains why the 1992 civil rights act was not called the Disabled Americans Act but the Americans with Disabilities Act.

Even if untrained in sign language, late-deafened people, too, will naturally develop a language of gestures. Although Mother is unwilling to go to sign-language classes, she and Dad have developed a repertoire of hand signals through which they communicate without her magic slate. Some of these are signs with which we all communicate (see Table 2.1). Others he has introduced after attending a few classes in signing. Still other gestures they have invented during their years of speechless communication. Back in 1892, baseball outfielder William "Dummy" Hoy, the major leagues' first deaf player, did the same when he enriched the game by inventing umpires' hand signals. With their colorful gestures for "Strike!" "Safe!" and "Yerr Out!" umpires could communicate with Hoy. Of course, such gestures communicate to fans as well—as referees now do through signs invented for all the major sports, whose fans are fluent in sports sign language.

Indeed, reports psychologist Robert Pollard, it was the naturalness of signed communication among the deaf that a hundred years ago led fifty-one of the sixty-one public schools for the deaf in America to teach in sign language—while their European counterparts were using oral methodologies. Deaf students' natural affinity for signing helped spread American sign language. Although

TABLE 2.1 Common Gestures

Message	*Gesture*
Stop	Hand raised, palm facing outward
Come here	Hand raised, palm inward, index finger waving
Quiet	Forefinger to lips
Stand up	Open palms of both hands motioning upward
Money	Rubbing together of thumb and first two fingers
What time?	Tapping of watch, raised eyebrows
Mediocre	Waggling of extended hands, showing both sides
Like a drink?	Hand around phantom glass to mouth
Good/bad	Thumb up/down

U.S. schools for the deaf reverted to oral methods for much of this century, the 1965 publication of William Stokoe's *Dictionary of American Sign Language* helped educators see that ASL is not a crude visual miming but a genuine and rich language for communicating and teaching.

Worshiping in Silence 27 NOVEMBER 1992

I neglected to bring my aid to Thanksgiving worship at our church yesterday. (Seldom do I need it at worship, given the already amplified sound. Moreover, the aid, overloaded by the powerful organ, transforms its music into a mush of noise.) But yesterday's experience confirmed that the march from sound toward silence is continuing. In accordance with tradition, people rose from their seats to offer spontaneous statements of thanksgiving. Sitting more or less in the middle of the 125 people, I soon noticed that I was hearing less than ever. So, pretending I was taking minutes, I entertained myself by counting the number of people whose statements I heard well enough to report on. Of the twenty-two people who spoke, I sufficiently discerned the words of only five. Carol, beside me, later acknowledged hearing most of what I had missed. Nevertheless, Carol reminded me, there is a point to my being there. One needn't hear to worship.

What Will People Think? 28 DECEMBER 1992

I've just completed a skin cancer prevention treatment that, for nearly three weeks, left my forehead a reasonable approximation of salsa sauce. Knowing that my appearance would be as unsightly as that of an adolescent with severe acne, I wondered how people would react, and how *I* would cope with going about in public—breakfasting in restaurants, teaching, speaking to a hundred people at a local church.

People did occasionally stare or ask what the problem was. Children were the most unabashed. But mostly, caught up in their own worlds, people didn't much seem to care. All of us are so busy worrying about ourselves that we're much less conscious of someone else's condition than we are of our own. And in less time than I expected, I adapted, too. You can't wallow in self-consciousness for long. Once you're engaged in reading or talking, your attention shifts to the subject or the person at hand and away from your face—which you can't see anyway.

What is true of the face is still truer of the ear. Who cares that I have any object (short of a banana) in my ear? Having coped with a "spaghetti face" (to use one of my kid's teasing descriptions) and having scanned a book containing photos of children who have learned to cope with severely malformed faces, I find the aid protruding from my ear a small price to pay for hearing. Indeed, as being hearing-impaired becomes part of my public identity (with the hearing aid bearing witness), it feels more and more natural and less and less like something to feel shame over.

To get past vain self-consciousness, we need to complete our graduation from adolescence. As teens become increasingly capable of thinking about their own thinking, and of thinking about what other people are thinking, they begin imagining what other people are thinking about *them.* Adolescence is therefore a time of amplified self-consciousness, as teens worry about how they look to others, without fully realizing that few care, because they're all focused on how *they* look to others. In one of his columns, Dave Barry recalls what it felt like:

> When my dad pulled up, wearing his poodle hat and driving his Nash Metropolitan—a comically tiny vehicle resembling those cars outside supermarkets that go up and down when you put in a quarter, except the Metropolitan looked sillier and had a smaller motor—I was mortified. I might as well have been getting picked up by a flying saucer piloted by some bizarre multi-tentacled stalk-eyed slobber-mouthed alien being that had somehow got hold of a Russian hat. I was horrified at what my peers might think of my dad; it never occurred to me that my peers didn't even notice my dad, because they were too busy being mortified by THEIR parents.
>
> Of course eventually my father stopped being a hideous embarrassment to me, and I, grasping the Torch of Dorkhood, became a hideous embarrassment to my son.

As we reach maturity, our concern for what others think subsides but never disappears, as plastic surgeons catering to people in midlife know well. Nor would we wish to become insensitive to others' reactions. We are, after all, social animals living in community. Still, captives though we are to vanity, we should pause to remember that others really don't care whether we have visible prostheses for our eyes or ears, and that our hearing loss may, unknown to us, be more conspicuous than any hearing aid.

A clever recent study revealed the extent to which we imagine that others notice us more than they do. Thomas Gilovich demonstrated a "spotlight effect" by having individual Cornell University students don Barry Manilow

T-shirts before entering a room with other students. Feeling self-conscious, the T-shirt–wearers guessed that nearly half of their peers would take note of the shirt as they walked in. In reality, only 23 percent did. I guess the moral is—whether you're wearing the wrong clothes or a hearing aid—relax. Fewer people notice than we imagine.

Interaction 7 JANUARY 1993

Our men's basketball coach stopped me yesterday evening to tease me about my interaction with his daughter's boyfriend from another college. At halftime she and he had come to an aisle near where a friend and I were seated. According to our coach's retelling of the incident, the boyfriend was enjoying meeting these two professors, whose work he had read. But my part in the conversation ended abruptly when I was handed the halftime statistics.

I admit that columnist Dave Barry may have been on to something in advising women to give up expecting sensitivity from some men: "If you were to probe deep inside the guy psyche, beneath that macho exterior and endless droning about things like the 1978 World Series, you would find, deep down inside, a passionate heartfelt interest in: the 1978 World Series." Before a game with our archrival, I once wondered aloud to Carol (who couldn't care less) why beating them was so important. "It isn't," she replied; "it doesn't matter. Compared to almost anything else, it's unimportant." "Oh, but it is important," I replied. "I'm just trying to figure out why."

But in this instance, there was more at issue than my

love of basketball and my identification with my school. Because I don't wear my hearing aid in noisy settings such as the basketball arena, *I couldn't hear those two.* Contrary to their impression, I was never a participant in their conversation with my friend.

The incident brings to mind other occasions where people have told me (unaware of my hearing loss) that they have tried and failed to get my attention. I wonder, How many people have I unknowingly offended? How many people have wrongly assumed that a person was uninterested, preoccupied, or ignoring them, rather than hard of hearing?

One Body, Many Parts 12 JANUARY 1993

Yesterday afternoon I found myself in a situation that was at once poignant and amusing. Louise, our blind director of Disabled Student Services, and her Seeing Eye dog came to my office with Chris, a student whose severe cerebral palsy prevents him from speaking or gesturing. By using his left big toe to operate a computer touchpad on his wheelchair, however, Chris can communicate. At least he can communicate to those who can understand the monotone computer voice. I couldn't (and Chris is my student in the new semester that starts today).

So there we sat in my office before visiting the classroom: Chris, who couldn't speak, Louise, who couldn't see, and Dave, who couldn't hear Chris. Yet thanks to Chris's and Dave's eyes and Louise's ears, the three of us managed, as an interdependent little group, to accomplish all our tasks. What St. Paul said of the church is true of any functioning group—it is like a body, with many complementary parts. One person is an eye, another an ear, another a toe—parts that support one another toward a common purpose. And so it was with our motley crew, as we wended our way down the hall and said good-bye.

3
Communication

To Wear or Not to Wear? 16 FEBRUARY 1993

A week ago, I was interviewed as Robert Schuller's guest at California's Crystal Cathedral, a worship service currently broadcast to twenty-three countries in Europe and around the globe via satellite. (More anxiety-producing for me than the viewing millions was my awareness that some people I know, including my family, would be in the television audience.) Should I wear my hearing aid or not?

I decided not to, partly because I was confident that, standing two feet from someone who was projecting to the 2,000 people in front of him, I'd have no trouble hearing—why not flow with the natural sound of his and my voices? Admittedly, though, after more than a year of public use the aid seldom comes to mind while I'm engaged in public dialogue. I therefore can't deny that the other factor in my decision was vanity—the desire not to *appear* infirm. This must be why I usually remove the aid when I'm having my picture taken. Usually, but not always: as "hearing-impaired" becomes more and more part of my public identity (as I disclose my difficulty and wear a visible aid), I find myself gradually becoming more comfortable with having people perceive me as I am.

My unaided conversation with Schuller before the services was a mild disaster. I missed the whole point of a story he told a couple of us about a fancy shirt he was wearing. And with my stress level noticeably rising, I missed or had to have him repeat several questions. Fortunately, his public voice was stronger than his offstage voice, so I survived the experience unscathed.

Conversation: A Two-Way Street 2 MARCH 1993

The question is often asked, Would you sooner give up seeing or hearing? A recent experience raised a corollary question. I took my student Chris, a fellow basketball fan, to our team's playoff game. The experience—ninety minutes in a car with someone who could hear but not speak—got me to thinking: Which is preferable—trying to relate to someone who cannot speak, or to someone who cannot hear?

Conversation is a two-way street. Chris, when deprived of his toe-operated computer, can receive but not send. The deaf, deprived of channels of unspoken communication, can send but not receive. Given a choice, would you sooner give up your ability to send or to receive messages? And which capacity would you more want your partner to have—the ability to hear you or to speak to you?

Signed Communication 15 MARCH 1993

This weekend I read Oliver Sacks' *Seeing Voices,* a sympathetic look at deaf culture, cognition, and communication. I learned some things I should have known:

American Sign Language originated in the early 1800s when the French Sign Language pioneer was invited to introduce Sign to America. The ASL which resulted combines French Sign Language with the preexisting American pidgin signs. Thus, to this day, people fluent in ASL have an easier time conversing in Sign with people in Paris than with people who speak most of the hundreds of other sign languages, including British Sign Language. Nevertheless, there is a universal enough grammar to the various sign languages that signers from different countries can usually establish communication much faster than can those who speak only their native language. When America's National Theatre of the Deaf visited their counterparts in Japan, the two groups were communicating fluently within hours.

Sign language waxed during the mid-1800s, and so did the educational achievements of those considered deaf and "dumb" (a word that in some cases carried the connotation of "stupid" as well as "mute"). Then, from the late 1800s until recently, sign language was suppressed in classrooms in favor of strenuous efforts to teach "oralism" (lipreading and speaking skills for the deaf). Sacks reports that these efforts had limited success and contributed to the deterioration in deaf students' educational progress. During the past two decades, as realization has grown that ASL is a genuine language that is readily and naturally grasped by deaf children, the pendulum has swung back toward signing (albeit often signed English in classrooms, rather than ASL).

Given the importance of language for thought, deaf children risk permanent retardation if they are not exposed to language—which, for them, means sign language—during their critical early years. "To be defective in language, for a human being, is one of the most desperate of calamities," notes Sacks, "for it is only through language that we enter fully into our human estate and culture, communicate freely with our fellows, acquire and share information. If we cannot do this, we will be bizarrely disabled and cut off—whatever our desires, or endeavors, or native capacities. And indeed, we may be so little able to realize our intellectual capacities as to appear mentally defective."

The life experience of the congenitally deaf (perhaps 250 thousand in this country) is so different from the experience of those among us who are hard of hearing and late-deafened that I do not pretend to imagine it. Yet there are points of overlap that make us, if not brothers and sisters, at least cousins. Sacks quotes Leo Jacobs' description (from *A Deaf Adult Speaks Out* [1980]) of the deaf person's sense of social estrangement: "You are left out of the dinner table conversation. It is called mental isolation. While everyone else is talking and laughing, you are as far away as a lone Arab on a desert that stretches along every horizon. . . . You thirst for connection. . . . You get the impression nobody understands or cares. . . . You are not granted even the illusion of participation."

A Special Bilingualism 17 MARCH 1993

Yesterday I had lunch with one of my better students, Letha, the child of deaf, signing parents. Although she has normal hearing, Letha is natively bilingual. Her first words were signed rather than spoken. Her mother's extended family—grandparents, aunts, uncles, cousins—are predominantly deaf, as are many of her family's friends, all of whom helped integrate Letha into a deaf culture. Sacks reports that among hearing people, those who, like Letha, have grown up in the deaf culture and have native competence in Sign are most readily welcomed as members of the deaf culture. Thus, in response to Letha's wondering whether she should consider a career that would harness her native understanding of the deaf, I remarked, "You have what so many others, try as they may, cannot gain—credibility and native fluency." She is, as she has written, "part of two different worlds: the hearing world and the deaf world."

Like many native signers, Letha didn't realize until a couple years ago that Sign is a complete language (or that, without studying another language, she had already met our college requirement for competence or coursework in a second language). Yet Letha and her hearing sister easily mix signing and speech in their conversations with each other and even prefer Sign for communicating silently or from a distance.

Sign is, of course, not one language but many, and Letha's family signs in a mix of signed English (a literal interpretation of English sentences, as currently used in many classes for the deaf and in the little signing box on a television screen) and ASL, a more expressive visual language with its own grammar. From Letha's demonstration of the two in class later, however, it was possible to detect words common to both.

Sounds Out of Focus 29 APRIL 1993

In *Deafness* (1969), David Wright observes, "The partially deaf, it seems to me, have the worst of both worlds. They hear enough to be distracted by noise yet not enough for it to be meaningful. . . . There is the strain of extracting significance from sounds that may be as loud as life yet out of focus; what comes through is an auditory fuzz."

What an apt metaphor—sounds out of focus, the auditory equivalent of a blurred picture. What is blurred, may not, however, seem blurred; rather, it seems merely unclear. When I'm driving, the sign down the road that I can't yet read doesn't look blurred; my eyes just can't yet read it. I become aware of my slightly inferior vision only when traveling with someone who can see better and thus read it sooner. Likewise, my moment-to-moment perception is that I'm hearing what is, as it is. I become aware that the sound is out of focus for me only when I'm with others who decipher what I miss.

Missing 10 JUNE 1993

Part-time hearing-aid use carries a risk. Those who never or always use their aid have it safely stored—in their dresser drawer or in their ear. Those of us who pop it in and out as the situation changes run a greater risk of losing it—as I did recently.

Because the carrying packet felt like too big a bulge in my pocket, I carried the little device—about the size of the end of my thumb—loose in my pocket, constantly checking to be sure it hadn't fallen out. Unfortunately, somewhere between a late morning meeting, where I used it, and bedtime, it disappeared—and about a thousand dollars with it.

On learning that I needed to be retested and refitted from scratch, I wondered how much my hearing would have declined in the nearly two years since the last testing. I had little doubt that my need for the aid was much greater than it had been two years ago. Then I had coped fine without it. While awaiting the replacement, I missed every fourth sentence during a committee meeting. I was, therefore, shocked when the audiologist tested me today and announced that my hearing was unchanged from the way it was nearly two years ago. What had changed was my awareness of how much I miss without the aid—that beastly little instrument that at first so irritated me.

Overcoming Conversational Exclusion 16 JUNE 1993

I write this five miles up in the air on my return flight from Seattle, where our extended family celebrated my son Peter's graduation from Seattle University. Sister Nancy's two hearing aids sit in the drawer, unused. Brother Dick three days earlier had gotten two new computer-assisted aids, and his are likely to fall into similar disuse—though not if his wife has any say in the matter.

With Mother, I communicate not only with her magic slate but also with my laptop computer, on which I can write ten times faster and with greater clarity. I write, then turn the screen to her. She replies, and so forth. We converse.

As part of our conversation, she tells me about the wonders of closed-captioned television. So I put what she's telling me in closed captions, and she is stunned when I turn the screen to reveal her own words.

Why doesn't someone invent what I've as yet been unable to find—a little two-screen typing device? The machine would look like a notebook computer, but it wouldn't require much computing power. It would require a second screen, though, with a remote cord that would allow the deaf person across the table, or even across the room, to view in real time what the other person is typing. It would open up possibilities for more fluid and complete conversation with nonsigning, late-deafened persons. And in gatherings of friends or family it would even allow a spouse or friend to close-caption group conversation (albeit in a simplified form).

What a wonderful thing this would be! Not to hear is to be socially excluded. Others' smiles and laughter tell the nonhearing person that something pleasant is happening—something he or she can't share. Given the importance of what we social psychologists call social comparison—calibrating our own experiences to what others are experiencing—it is understandable why Mother doesn't relish staying late at parties.

Never Giving Up 14 AUGUST 1993

Hope still springs. Two studies reported in *Science* have now stimulated the regeneration of hair cells in mammals. In live guinea pigs, and in test-tube samples of the human ear, investigators managed by chemical means to trick tissue into growing new, though immature, hair cells. The researchers are a long way from applying the research to human beings. (For one thing, regenerated hair cells would have to connect to the auditory nervous system.) But as one researcher put it, except for the cochlear implant, "We're the only game in town. If you can't regenerate hair cells, there's little chance you will ever truly restore hearing for the seriously impaired or deaf."

Hidden Treasure 8 SEPTEMBER 1993

Discover magazine has just announced its 1993 technology awards, one of which went to Philips Hearing Instruments for the first "invisible" hearing aid. It's so tiny—half an inch long—that it fits deep in the auditory canal. The aid is not only cosmetically pleasing (who among us is without vanity?), but auditorily better. It delivers the sound right to the eardrum, doesn't turn breezes into blizzards, and needn't be removed when the wearer is talking on the phone. When it comes out in a version that amplifies only the sounds I need, I'll be a customer.

"This Is Your Captain Speaking" 21 NOVEMBER 1993

Airplanes are one place where poor hearing is a blessing. Without a hearing aid, the plane's roar is mere white noise—a not-bad background for uninterrupted concentration on work. But then come the unexpected words from the cockpit, which go right past me without my knowing what has been said. My experience must be akin to that of non-English-speaking persons who wish they could understand the description of the part of the country they are flying over, the news of when they will be landing, the announcement of what the weather will be—and who may wonder if they have missed more important information, about turbulence up ahead or a flight delay. Other announcements over a public-address system can also be a problem for the hard of hearing because they are often some distance away from the speaker and are fighting background noise. Although the people who design public address systems can't hope to enable communication with those who are most severely impaired, they might want to test, under realistic conditions, a sampling of the legions of the mildly impaired. If they did, I suspect they'd be surprised at how many people just don't get it.

Listening to Enya 10 DECEMBER 1993

My daughter Laura introduced me to an Irish folksinger, Enya. Rarely do I enjoy my children's music, but Enya's enchanting voice falls into that narrow zone where our tastes overlap. The rich rhythms of one particular song stir my emotions. Unable to decipher more than a word here and there, I play and replay one song dozens of times on the car stereo over a period of weeks. Gradually, I infer that she is expressing ideas I want to hear, beckoning us to create a more just and peaceful world.

If only I could make out the lyrics, I would enjoy the song even more. The packaging includes no transcription for this song. So I ask Laura to listen with me to the song on C.D. and dictate the words to me. Somehow, Laura's ears decipher what mine, at any volume, cannot. What is humming to me is oddly clear to her.

And the words? I wasn't even close. The song expresses a soulful longing to rejoin a lover far across the ocean.

On another occasion I had been enjoying a Celtic music C.D. for some weeks, until Carol walked into the living room one late February day and wondered why I was still listening to Christmas music. Christmas music? I had no idea what the lyrics were, but I liked what the music evoked in me. Vocal music apparently is for me what a Latin Mass is to a lover of classical choral music—something that works nonverbally.

Loving Being Deaf? 18 DECEMBER 1993

Letha, my student fluent in Sign, dropped around with the October issue of *Deaf Michigander*, which her mother thought I might enjoy. Three things catch my eye.

One is an ad from a Detroit-area optometry firm that features ASL-trained staff and doctors. "At 1st Optometry, you won't have to bring pencil & paper at all!" I'm impressed, but also curious: Assuming that these people are mostly hearing (how could they interact with the general public, if not?), what motivated them to learn Sign? Are they, like Letha, native signers? If they learned Sign late, how fluent are they? Are they like travelers who, by dusting off their college Spanish when visiting Mexico, can awkwardly communicate the basics but not much more?

Second, an educated letter writer offers kudos to this new newspaper and its twenty-one-year-old publisher, along with a word of concern: "From time to time there will be a grammatical error or a spelling error in the *Deaf Michigander*. . . . I strongly recommend that someone proofread the *Deaf Michigander* before it goes to print." The publisher's reply: "Yes, we are aware that every issues are not proofread thoroughly." Elsewhere, the publisher reports on his search for subscribers: "It should not be a problem reaching out at least 1,000 people during the first year to break it even." Would I be right to assume that the natively deaf young publisher lacks a mastery of English grammar?

Third, a photo features a button that reads: "I love being deaf!" Although I can't help admiring the positive spirit, I have trouble empathizing. I hope to be able to say, "I love being me" or "I love life"—even though I'm deaf. But could I ever say I love the deafness? Not after knowing what it's like to hear. Yes, there's much more to life than hearing. But surely, just as seeing is better than blindness, so hearing is better than deafness. Only a person who has no clue about what vision is could say that blindness is better, and that the Creator goofed in giving us five senses. "C'mon guys," I think. "You needn't demean the world you've never known in order to celebrate the integrity of sign language, the abilities of deaf people, or the rights of deaf workers." Or am I overinterpreting the button, which may only be meant to say, "I accept and affirm who I am, as I am," in which case I applaud the statement.

The Silent Sound of One's Own Voice 3 JANUARY 1993

We've just returned from our second Christmas out west in twenty-six years. The completeness of Mother's deafness was evident one evening when the rest of us were talking. She thought she was turning the television sound to "mute," but unknowingly, she had turned *off* the muting and thus blasting the rest of us with sound that she couldn't hear.

Despite her deafness, she talks pretty well (although occasionally too loudly in social settings). So I ask her: "How are you able to speak at the appropriate volume? Can you hear yourself?"

Curiously, she doesn't really know how she does it. She surely doesn't "hear" her voice through her ears, but she apparently can feel it from inside. Perhaps a lifetime of talking experience, combined with occasional feedback when she's too loud or soft, enables her to control the muscular effort. Still, I wonder, what is the sound of silence? What is it like to speak and not hear oneself? Is it rather like the silence we hearing people can experience when we plug our ears and whisper?

Never Too Late to Learn 7 FEBRUARY 1994

Yesterday's *New York Times* had a story about Junius Wilson, a deaf man who was jailed in 1925 on a charge of attempted rape, declared insane, and sent to North Carolina's mental hospital for blacks, where he was castrated. Although the charges were dropped in the 1970s, Wilson, was not freed—until last Friday, when at age ninety-six he was released to live in a cottage on the hospital grounds.

Now for the rest of the story. Another elderly deaf man visited Wilson, and they communicated in the old "Raleigh Sign," a form of sign language once taught to blacks. But the line that caught my eye: "Mr. Wilson is being taught American Sign Language." At ninety-six? Folk wisdom admonishes us that old dogs can't learn new tricks. But it also tells us that you're never too old to learn. We know that Wilson is too old to learn the tricks of ASL grammar (few adults of any age can master the subtle grammar of a new language). But he, and late-deafened people as well, can surely learn some basic ASL vocabulary (much as adult immigrants to this country often learn a rudimentary English that enables them to negotiate the culture). At ninety-six, Junius Wilson has at last been freed from his hospital cell. Perhaps by the time he's a hundred, Wilson will be freer, too, to communicate with others.

Finding Ways to Communicate 8 MARCH 1994

During another recent visit to Seattle, I came to realize that Mother actually knows three dozen or so common ASL signs, plus a few that she and Dad have invented for themselves. She knows them because Dad learned them at a class and from a video and began introducing them into conversation.

But of course! I suddenly realized. Late-deafened people's learning of sign language needn't take place in class (helpful though that might be). It is necessary only that their partners learn signing and use it while speaking. In this way the partner (or a child or other significant person) becomes the teacher. The deaf person doesn't need Sign to speak to the partner; it's the other way around.

Will I ever use Sign (at best a pidgin sign language of mostly nouns and verbs)? That will depend, first, on how long I live and how complete a hearing loss I sustain. But it will also depend on whether Carol or any others close to me also learn and use signs.

Political Correctness, or Sensitivity to Others' Feelings? 1 MAY 1994

The terminology we use to refer to the hearing-impaired may change sooner than later. The International Federation of Hard of Hearing People and the World Federation of the Deaf agree: neither likes the term "hearing-impaired." In 1991 they jointly agreed that "'hearing impaired' is a term intended to cover deaf and hard of hearing individuals under a single category. However, deaf and hard of hearing persons in most countries reject this definition because it fails to recognize any distinction differentiating these two social categories" (www.ifhoh. org). If it's not insensitive (by current standards of political correctness) to refer to people as "deaf" or "nonhearing" (or white or blue-eyed), then what is insensitive about saying that people are "hearing-impaired"? As one such person, I don't feel the slight. But language usage and sensitivities have a way of changing. Perhaps by the time you read this, some part of the terminology used here will seem inappropriate (as each generation's does to the next).

I Know My Answer, but What Is the Question? 12 JUNE 1994

A person laughs, while empathizing, with the trials of others with hearing loss, such as "Tomato Face" in today's Ann Landers column:

> Dear Ann Landers: I have been going with a wonderful man for two years. We get along beautifully, and my family is crazy about him. He speaks softly and has a well-modulated voice, which is the problem. My hearing is not 100 percent, and I am too embarrassed to ask him to keep repeating things.
>
> Last night, I think he asked me to marry him, but I'm not sure. What should I do?—TOMATO FACE
>
> Dear Face: If he's serious, he'll ask again. Meanwhile, get your hearing checked. Heaven knows what else you've been missing.

Penetrating the Lonely Silence 25 AUGUST 1994

I've just returned from another trip to Seattle, where, armed with a new laptop computer, I had the best conversations with Mother that I've had in years. When I sat beside her and instructed the computer to display typed dialogue in large, easy-to-read type, she could follow easily. Moreover, once she was in better touch with the outside world, her personality seemed to perk up. Surely, I think, someone should soon be producing that dual-screen device that would allow me to see what I'm typing while allowing her to read my closed-captioning of family conversation as it occurs.

4

Support

Joining a Self-Help Group 13 SEPTEMBER 1994

I have just corresponded with, and joined, Self Help for Hard of Hearing People (SHHH, at www.shhh.org), a national organization offering resources and support to "people with hearing loss." (The editor of SHHH publications writes that they use this term out of respect for those within deaf culture who take offense at the implication that the deaf have an impairment.) The organization offers what looks to be a wonderful smorgasbord of low-cost publications dealing with hearing loss, its emotional consequences, communication devices, and the education of children with hearing loss.

Facing the Truth 13 OCTOBER 1994

An acquaintance—a pastor in her late forties—called the other day seeking advice, because she was ready to "come out" as hard of hearing and be fitted with aids. "Let me guess," I said. "Your husband has been pestering you endlessly. Your family complains about your having the television too loud. You find yourself missing more, and frustrated by it."

"Yes, yes, yes," she replied sheepishly, as if I had been spying on her home life. My own experience has so often been confirmed by others' tales that I think I could write their stories. Hearing loss is in one sense like alcoholism: family members detect the problem sooner and see it as more serious than do the afflicted, who deny that the problem is really so bad. Moreover, unlike arthritis and other physical disorders, hearing loss is painless (physically painless, that is). And because our hearing at some frequencies may remain intact, we rebut family criticism with protestations like "How can I have a hearing problem if I can hear the timer on the microwave when you can't?" (For most people, it's actually low-frequency sounds—those of a rumbling train or distant thunder—that continue to come in clearly.) No wonder one source reports an average delay between the onset of hearing loss and the recourse to professional evaluation as six years.

Eventually, however, the combined effect of frustration and family members' persistence wears down the denial. My pastor-friend, finding herself missing more than half of what her parishioners were saying at a morning prayer group, finally had to agree with her husband: Yes, there is a problem, and it is necessary to do something about it.

I also ventured a prediction: "When you get the hearing aid you will hate it at first. Oh, you'll like hearing—but you'll dislike all the extraneous, distracting noise, including the altered feedback of your own voice and the self-consciousness it triggers. It is like adjusting to new glasses, only it takes longer."

A Missed Good-bye 29 OCTOBER 1994

Carol arose early yesterday to catch a plane for an East Coast meeting. So I got up early, too, and waited to see her off. As she finished packing, I sat in the family room, taking a look at the previous day's paper. She came down to the adjacent kitchen, then seemed to go back upstairs.

After ten more minutes I noticed that it was past the time when she had wanted to leave, so I called up the stairs to let her know. When silence greeted my call, I checked the garage and found she had left. Left without even saying good-bye, after I had gotten up and then sat downstairs waiting to send her off with a kiss!

When she called the next evening, I chided her for walking out on her dutiful mate. "Not so," she replied. "I gathered my things and said good-bye, and you just sat there with your nose in the paper, ignoring me. So I left."

We laughed, but I couldn't resist admonishing her again, with tongue half in cheek: "As time goes on, you're going to have to become more sensitive to the world of the auditorily disadvantaged."

A Written Message via Telephone 3 NOVEMBER 1994

Today here in Seattle Dad explained that Mother wouldn't be joining us at worship on Sunday. "She won't go places where she might meet someone she used to know. She's afraid someone might try to talk to her and think she is stupid." The misperception that the deaf are dumb has, of course, been the bane of many deaf people who have been wrongly judged to be retarded. Sometimes, though, as in this instance, I suspect, a self-conscious person misperceives a misperception. (In my 11 July 1992 entry I described how people, when they are conscious of being different, may misinterpret others' innocent behavior.)

At eighty-five, Mother is about to get—as a result of my father's initiative—a text telephone (called a TTY, after the old teletypewriter, or also a telecommunication device for the deaf, or TDD). After receiving $325 from Dad, the state health department will bring over a display screen (on which a blinking red light indicates a call). The phone company, thanks to a modest tax paid by all telephone customers, then will provide a transcription of callers' words, to which Mother will make a spoken reply. Family members have suggested, half jokingly, "Gee, Dad, you should get two phone lines. Then, when we visit, we could use one to call Mother on the other." (Of course, the portable, dual-screen computer I envision would make the same result possible.)

Hearing Lost, Conversation Lost 31 DECEMBER 1994

The initial TTY installation has not been a resounding success, for a reason that illustrates the social consequences of deafness. Mother has been out of the conversational loop for so long, living essentially alone in her silent world, that she now finds TTY-assisted conversation difficult. Family callers ask questions, and she responds with Yes,

No, or an answer so terse that the conversation goes dead until the caller can think of what to say next. Dad has already replaced the initial machine with a new one, with a bigger display. He hopes this will engage her more fully as she learns to cope with the device (much as she already has adjusted to brief conversations assisted by a writing board or a magic pad).

An Unwanted Earplug 15 JANUARY 1995

Last weekend in Del Mar, California, where I'd gone for a publisher's sales meeting, my hearing aid became plugged with wax and stopped functioning. You might think that someone who has come to depend on the aid would notice when it was off. But when the room is noisy and your attention is focused on something, the defective aid can act instead as an earplug.

That was my experience Saturday night (at a party celebrating a milestone for *Psychology* sales). Owing partly to the din of conversation, and partly to one plugged ear, I missed much of what people were saying to me—and had to make the usual split-second decisions about whether to acknowledge an unheard comment with a smile or ask to have it repeated, if the context seemed to indicate that it was important.

A Cochlear-Implant Success Story 2 FEBRUARY 1995

The February issue of the *SHHH Journal* offered former director Rocky Stone's report on his new cochlear implant. I was amazed. Having become deaf and then having lost his ability to lip-read because of deteriorating vision, he had become "unable to access information or to communicate effectively with anyone including my family." The implant surgery took place in July, and a month later he was tested and hooked up to a speech-processor program. Four days later

> our son had a family gathering to celebrate the success of my operation. There were 16 people present, five of them were children screaming like banshees. The other 11 were one-on-one conversations, which created an atmosphere with considerable background noise. Previously, under these circumstances, I would simply say hello to everyone and, at the first possibility, slip into another room and watch the TV in silence and isolation.
>
> On this day, however, with all the conversations going on around me, with the children shouting and playing, I did not ask that they be silenced, I did not move into another room. I stood with my son-in-law and listened for 30 minutes in a conversation and did very well. I then had conversations with each of the other adults, and heard what they all said. . . .
>
> On the eighth day after [I had received] the speech processor, the phone rang and I was alone. I thought, well, I'll take a chance. So, I answered the phone and recognized the voice of Betsy Bomberg, my audiologist in New York. We had a wonderful conversation. She was astonished . . . happy . . . even joyful. And I reciprocated those feelings.

How fortunate for Rocky Stone and for all of us who are hard of hearing that we are alive today. Twenty years ago there were not only no cochlear implants, but

no closed captioning
no telephones with volume control

no telephone relay services
no digital hearing aids
no F.M. systems in other public places
no Americans with Disabilities Act

Left Out 9 FEBRUARY 1995

Yesterday evening, as Carol laid out some things for me to give our parents while I was on a speaking trip to the Seattle area, she wondered aloud whether we would ever feel regret or guilt over the things we were too busy to do for our parents, "like your writing to your mother instead of just sending tapes to your father."

Thirty-some years ago, when my parents could both hear, I promised to send as a Christmas gift a cassette voice letter every two or three weeks for the next year. My father, who would return the tape with his own news from home, so obviously appreciated this that I have continued sending the cassettes up to the present. He calls them the best gift I could ever give him ("You just don't know how much it means to us").

But of course Mother long ago ceased hearing this news. For a time she relied on my father's spoken summaries, and now she reads his written notes. She is left out of the direct communication loop, apart from occasional clippings, children's reports, and brief notes we direct to them both (and so far she hasn't really taken to TTY communication). "I guess you're not very sensitive to the hearing-impaired," said Carol with a smirk. And I couldn't deny it.

Missing Out on Family Fun 12 FEBRUARY 1995

Upon hearing Mother describe her sense of isolation in the midst of hearing people, my sister Nancy exclaimed, "I know how that feels! When I visit [my daughter] Kathleen and her in-laws in Sweden, I can take being the odd person out of the conversation for only so long before saying, 'Kathleen, translate for me!'—like Dad writing for Mother on the magic slate. But then Kathleen gets involved and forgets, and before long I get up and see if there are dishes to do."

Yes, I think: I, too, occasionally had that feeling of being left out during an academic sojourn in Germany. And it *is* like the feeling you have when you can't hear the things everyone else does.

Reading John Hull's *Touching the Rock: An Experience of Blindness* (1990) further helps me understand why Mother could want to leave family gatherings early, frustrating the rest of us in the process, for we valued our parents' presence and delighted in Dad's obvious enjoyment at having his family gathered together. Hull recalls an occasion when a friend brought over some late Christmas presents, which his children were relishing. As the friend played happily and imaginatively with Hull's children, pointing things out and looking through books with them, Hull fell into a funk. He reported that it made him "more sharply aware of my own difficulties in playing with the children. . . . I hear the children and everyone else whooping with delight [much as Mother *sees* but cannot *hear* our own family fun], making comments, and it is as if the knowledge which I do have mocks the knowledge which I don't have, while the poignancy of that contrast makes me want to have no more knowledge at all." After retreating to his office, Hull recalls feeling no sadness, bitterness, or anger. He feels, rather, "a sort of numbness of recoil."

Can She Really Hear Sometimes? 12 FEBRUARY 1995

During the visit home, Mother explained how, although she is deaf, she will on rare occasions hear something. That's strange, I think. She is so deaf she cannot hear me clap beside her ear. So how, with the total nerve deafness brought on by the atrophy of her cochlear hair-cell receptors, could she ever hear?

Auditory hallucinations are one obvious possibility. Another explanation came up at the dinner table. "Earlier, I heard David say, 'My battery went dead,'" Mother stated. But her recollection illustrates what research psychologists know as memory construction. No one else around the table had heard those words, because I *typed* them on the laptop computer I was using to talk with her—and noted her comprehending nod as she *read* the words.

Living with Criticism 5 MARCH 1995

An article in today's *USA Weekend* Sunday supplement describes the tribulations of Heather Whitestone, this year's Miss America. As a deaf person who lost 95 percent of her hearing when she was eighteen months old, she learned, while growing up in a hearing family and school system, to read lips and to speak English. As an adolescent, she also learned to sign, which she reportedly did flawlessly when signing the national anthem for 120 million viewers of the recent Super Bowl game.

Although she has been celebrated as an inspirational example and is admired for her motto, "Anything is Possible," she illustrates two points mentioned earlier. First, a person who learns any language after childhood usually will not perfectly master its grammar and syntax. "She's a sweet human being," reports Gallaudet University campus relations director Sherry Dubon. "And yes, she signed. But her signing skills show she was brought up in a hearing environment. She's not fluent, in other words."

Second, her lipreading and speaking have angered deaf culture advocates, who don't welcome having a person who can speak being viewed as their representative to the hearing world. "I never imagined becoming Miss America would throw me into a communications war," she says. "I feel caught between the hearing and deaf worlds. It's been very frightening." Before the pageant, she reportedly had little contact with anyone, deaf or hearing, outside her little Alabama town. But she now advocates "whatever communication option" works best for a person, and she is learning to live with the criticism. "I've decided to be true to myself. I want to feel comfortable with myself. I am comfortable speaking. I am comfortable in my own voice." With those words, she does speak for many of us.

5
Aids and Advice

A Failed Experiment 9 MARCH 1995

The TTY experiment has ended, in failure. "I thought it would be a great idea," said Dad on his most recent tape. "But if she doesn't want to talk to people, I guess I shouldn't make her." After nine years of not conversing, and at eighty-five, she finds new ways of communicating hard to cope with. "I am still learning," said Michelangelo at eighty-five. But Michelangelo wasn't learning a new way of relating to people.

Feeling Like a Fool 22 MAY 1995

Not hearing can be embarrassing. This weekend, I began my participation in a White House character education conference with a sex education task force meeting. The chairperson, sitting immediately to my left, introduced the meeting, and I heard him thank me for my support in helping underwrite the conference. Then, while the CNN camera was rolling, I noticed the room go silent and saw the person beside me wave his finger a few times. Finally, he leaned over and said, "We're supposed to introduce ourselves," whereupon I realized that the CNN camera and microphone were pointed at me, as the first person in the circle. Throughout the conference I managed to sit in the first row (even for an hourlong session with President Clinton), yet I was unable to hear most audience questions and comments.

En route home from the airport I honked at a car stopped in front of me after a light had turned green. I was oblivious to what this driver had heard—an oncoming ambulance, whose siren penetrated my ears moments later just before it crossed in front of us. "Just what I worry about," Carol later remarked, reminding me of her concerns about my listening to music while driving. To be hard of hearing is sometimes to look and feel like a fool.

The Ever-Present Decision 26 JUNE 1995

I face a repeat of the 16 February 1993 question: Do I or don't I wear my very visible hearing aid during a national television taping session (for an NBC documentary on happiness). I expect to have no difficulty hearing interviewer Maria Shriver, with her sharp, clear voice, or my big-voiced fellow interviewee, happiness researcher Ed Diener. This time, not wishing to seem ashamed, I do wear it. Curiously, the producer, having surely noticed the blocky aid, points me to a seat that most visibly displays that side of my face. Does she want to make a statement?

I almost didn't have to make the choice. Three weeks before, I put some clothes through the washer and dryer with the hearing aid still in a pocket. The bad news: it had to be sent in for repair. The good news: it was very clean. Part of me was hoping it would *not* be returned in time for the interview, so that I could evade the issue of whether to wear it, but I had no such luck. In the intervening time, however, I could have used it on a five-day speaking trip to Hong Kong. Following the group conversations in restaurants, in Chinese-accented English, was particularly stressful.

Lip-Synching, Finger-Synching? 23 OCTOBER 1995

Last week Carol and I listened to a few minutes of a New York Philharmonic concert on PBS. As the conductor launched into the next piece, the camera panned to the low-frequency oboes, which seemed resistant to the conductor's gesticulations with the baton. The camera then returned to the conductor, who was now waving his arms yet more energetically, still without any audible response from the orchestra.

I turned to Carol, who assured me that the orchestra *was* playing. Still hearing nothing, I amused myself by imagining that the Philharmonic was having a labor dispute, a work stoppage. The oboe section, I mused, was playing as my older son once admitted to doing: as he marched with his elementary school band, he fingered his saxophone to simulate playing but, distrusting his own music, didn't blow into the instrument.

Breakthrough! 20 NOVEMBER 1995

To readers in the future, what I am about to describe may seem mundane. But from the vantage point of the present, "exciting" strikes me as inadequate to describe what I've recently been discovering. It started a few weeks back when I stumbled across the Gallaudet University Technology Assessment Center on the World Wide Web. I wrote to ask whether the personnel knew of any computer technology that would facilitate communication with such people as my mother by visually displaying spoken words. Gallaudet responded in the negative, so I forgot about the idea until Carol happened on a new IBM advertisement for voice-dictation software that claims to do precisely that. I e-mailed IBM about possible adaptation of their technology to the needs of the deaf and got a response suggesting that they weren't yet thinking about that market.

Then my son Andy alerted me to two competing systems, each of which, like the IBM system, he has now explored through the Web and ordered for testing. The IBM product has arrived, and it is impressive. After a two-hour enrollment period, during which the computer learns the user's voice patterns, it is possible to speak at up to a hundred words a minute (with breaks between words) and then see those words appear with remarkable accuracy on the computer screen.

What a godsend this would be for my parents! We're thinking about putting together a special Christmas present for them from all their children. The package would include a computer that could also be used for e-mail, a large monitor to display the spoken words, the best available voice-translation software, and software designed by

Andy to make it all ultra-simple for older people to learn. They would just turn on the computer, click on an icon for voice translation, start talking, and watch as large type spilled across the screen.

Ideally, the small computer would be left on continually in the living room, so that it would be instantly available. Other family members could also take advantage of it. I described the idea to Dick, and his immediate response was that it would be "phenomenal"—a gift he is sure our other siblings would want to collaborate on.

Andy and I have been speculating whether other non-signing deaf people and their families would also benefit from such an innovation. Surfing the Web again—where I discovered a whole panoply of information and forums enabling the deaf to communicate with one another—I gleaned this statistic from a Gallaudet page on demography. The National Center for Health Statistics estimated in 1991 that 1.15 million people "at best, can hear and understand words shouted in the better ear." Of those, 72 percent—830 thousand—are older people who were deafened late in life. Those 830 thousand people constitute the potential beneficiaries of such technology. (But surely, given all the professionals working with the deaf and all the university centers for research on audiology and deafness, others must already be thinking along these lines.)

A Very Special Gift 29 FEBRUARY 1996

With Andy's considerable help, we did assemble a family Christmas package, including a computer with Pentium processor and sound card, Windows 95, and DragonDictate. Andy created a friendly interface to facilitate Dad's use, including a ninety-picture family slide show as a screen saver, and delivered it in mid-January. After three hours of use, I found myself able to speak to Mother at nearly a hundred words a minute, with about 95 percent recognition accuracy (that is, the program made no more errors than I make in typing). Moreover, it can make sense of grammar and correctly spells sentences such as "Their house is over there" and "Give two cookies to her, too."

If you make a mistake or misspeak a word, just say, "Scratch that," and it's gone. If the program "hears" a word wrong and it needs correction, you just say, "Oops," and it offers you a menu of alternate choices or allows you to type in the correct word.

For my eighty-seven-year-old dad, the learning curve is slower (slow enough that it's hard to see how the device could be commercially viable for computer-illiterate octagenarians just yet, unless they had extensive tutoring). But with patient instruction from Andy, followed by a visit from me, Dad has caught on and is using the system both to dictate messages to his children and grandchildren via e-mail and to tell Mother much more than the magic slate permits. "As you can guess, I am beginning to understand how to use the dictation mode," he explained via e-mail shortly after my visit. "I can move along fairly rapidly and do not have to make many corrections. Again, I say thanks for what you and the rest did in giving and pushing me into a new pleasure of my life."

The world should know about this new capability—and surely soon it will. As performance improves and costs fall, its practicality for communicating with the deaf, and the advantages it offers to those who are paralyzed, will surely increase.

Mishearing 6 SEPTEMBER 1996

My hearing aid is in the shop again, and Carol occasionally becomes exasperated when I don't hear her aright. Sometimes, however, the results are hilarious (to others, at least). At a recent family gathering I was stunned to hear my sister say, "I had a picture of an autopsy blown up." "You enlarged a picture of what?" I queried. She repeated more slowly: "Of an autumn scene."

It's an experience common to the hard of hearing. In the most recent issue of *Hearing Loss*, Pastor Mark Dill of Cumberland, Maryland, chortles over the phenomenon a psychologist might describe as the imposition of one's mental "set" on the perception of an equivocal stimulus. Given ambiguous visual or auditory information, the brain strains to find meaning.

> While preaching on Sunday morning, July 14, 1996, I was trying to involve the congregation in the sermon by asking a few questions. The first of those questions was, "How many of you write checks?"
>
> A woman seated near the back thought to herself, "I'm not going to raise my hand . . . that's none of his business!" A few people however did raise their hands, and she was wondering why.

"Come on now, be honest. How many of you write checks?"

This time most of the people in the congregation raised their hands. But not the woman near the back. The woman's husband nudged her and said to her, "Go ahead, raise your hand." But she just glared at him with a wrinkled brow and a cold stare.

Later that afternoon when she and her husband were discussing the sermon at home she finally admitted for the first time that she might need to think about getting a hearing aid. After all, she thought the question I had asked was, "How many of you like sex?"

What Am I Missing? 28 NOVEMBER 1996

This week while I was guest lecturing for a colleague who was away, I as usual welcomed student comments and questions. One young woman spoke so softly that even after moving as close as possible to her, I could catch only a few words. To help her understand that she needed to project to the whole class, I interrupted her (lest she infer from my hearing aid that the problem lay merely with my poor hearing) and turned to ask students across the room whether they could hear her, certain that they could not.

To my astonishment, the students farthest away all nodded—yes, they could hear what I could not. Feeling chagrined, I let her finish and *thought* I had caught the gist of her comment. Alas, my response must have indicated to the class that I had not understood her. For after I congratulated the next student on his cogent observation, he deflected the praise, saying that he was simply rearticulating for me the previous student's comment.

Should I Just Stay Home? 4 MAY 1997

Some recent experiences suggest an imperceptible yet insidious deterioration in my hearing.

Over the lunch hour I play pickup basketball without my hearing aid in. The other day my shot was twice blocked from behind by someone I didn't know was there. Not having heard him bearing down on me from behind, I chide my defender for wearing silencers on his shoes. When a friend later teased me about not having heard, I observed, "That must be what it's like for the Gallaudet University basketball team."

"Is the symphonette playing?" I asked yesterday as we marched into our community civic center for the Hope College commencement. "Sure," answered the colleague on my left. "Don't you hear it?"

"I don't hear a thing," I replied.

The previous week in church I had been perplexed when the bell choir stopped in the middle of a piece. Turning to look, I saw that the ringers were, in fact, swinging the big (low-tone) bells—with no discernible result. I whispered my perception of this curious phenomenon to Carol, who rolled her eyes and admonished me to put in my hearing aid.

Should I Go High-Tech? 29 AUGUST 1997

Sitting right in front at our opening convocation, no more than twenty feet from a colleague who was addressing an audience of nearly a thousand over the P.A. system, I could make out barely half his remarks. Such experiences, in combination with a letter from an audiologist alerting me to new digital hearing technology, drove me to make an appointment to be retested. Perhaps something better now exists.

When I went in for testing today, the audiologist discovered what it was I'd been feeling when trying to clear my right ear—a blockage of hardened wax. It took him ten minutes of working with different instruments to get it out . . . and to discover that it wasn't wax. It was the remnants of a wad of wet Kleenex I had stuck in there to block out the sound of a noisy air conditioner in a motel several months back. He grinned: "For three dollars, you know, you can buy earplugs that will do the same job more safely. They really work better."

After testing me, he told me again that there had been no significant change since three years ago. When I compared the charts, though, I could see that the right ear, formerly much better, had declined some, and he granted there had been a little slippage in the left ear, too. No matter, it will be years before I'm as deaf as a post. And in the meantime there's the new generation of digital aids, available in a less visible in-the-ear format or in a version that sits behind the ear. (Most people choose the latter, partly for reasons of cost). But his main point was that *two* inexpensive ($350) hearing aids would serve me better than one $1,400 high-tech aid.

After demonstrating the two aids, he removed them . . . and I had to ask him to speak up (will embarrassments never cease?). "Call me if you'd like to make an appointment to be fitted," he said. "Well," I replied, "I already know what my wife will say—what spouses always say, I suppose." He nodded and laughed.

During the demonstration I was not pleased to have the hiss of the air conditioning magnified. When I called the audiologist who originally fitted me with the high-tech hearing aid, he said that a new generation of fully digital (not just "digitally programmable") aids would become available that would, as I'd hoped, *not* amplify constant sound.

Weak Signals or Faulty Receivers? 16 SEPTEMBER 1997

Carol, arriving home after chairing a church board meeting, remarked that she tends not to participate in the time of free prayer, "because some people I can't hear, and I don't want to look stupid by repeating what someone has already said."

I smirk, and wonder aloud when *she* will have *her* hearing tested. She resists: "It's the way you say, dear. Some people just don't speak up."

I think of Carol later, when reading a *Reader's Digest* anecdote about a man who thought his wife was losing her hearing. To test it, he stood thirty feet behind her and asked, "Barbara can you hear me?" Hearing no response, he moved up to twenty feet behind her and repeated, "Barbara, can you hear me?" Still no reply. So he advanced to ten feet and asked, "Now can you hear me?" "Yes, dear," Barbara answered. "For the *third* time, *yes!*"

Carol's sheepish resistance also prompts a question: Might the mates of people who are significantly hard of hearing tend to perceive their own comparatively milder hearing loss as normal hearing? A mountain of research reveals that social comparisons control our judgments.

How we feel about our income, our grades, or our sex life depends on the comparisons we make with real and imagined others. How we evaluate our hearing surely does, too. In comparing themselves with a partner who has acute hearing, those with mild hearing loss may feel impaired. ("You hear a cat meowing? I don't!") By contrast, if they compare themselves with a partner who has significant hearing loss, they may feel thankful for their "good hearing" ("Listen—can't you hear the phone ringing?")

Is Digital the Way to Go? 28 SEPTEMBER 1997

Mark Ross, in the current issue of *Hearing Loss,* writes of the still-to-be-realized potential of digital hearing aids. Studies to date have not found them discernibly better than the best traditional (analog) aids. Users do seem to prefer them, but it will take a double-blind study (in which neither the audiologist nor the patient knows which type of aid is being tested) to determine whether patients' enthusiasm represents the old placebo effect. When people hear excited talk about a state-of-the-art computer hearing aid and, with high hopes and expectations, try it out, the testimonials are almost inevitably positive.

But Ross looks forward to the day when digital aids will transpose frequencies that users hear poorly into frequencies that they hear better. And why not? Like audio delivered by a desktop computer, the sound conveyed by the digital aid has simply been converted into discrete positive and negative charges, represented by a string of binary digits, such as 11011100; and that signal has then been transformed into the sound projected to my ear. So why not take the low voices I hear poorly and make them into higher-pitched voices that I could hear better? As my hearing worsens, I'd surely rather hear soft-spoken men sounding like men with high treble voices—or even like women—than not hear them at all.

And think of the possibilities that speech-recognition software offers. If digital sound processors can be "taught" to recognize words in natural, continuous speech (and as the success of DragonDictate indicates, that future is near at hand), then perhaps people who are severely hard of hearing could carry portable display devices (or wear displaying glasses). Like a teleprompter, such devices could display speech in captioned form. Given the rate at which this technology is developing, my fantasy is almost sure to become reality by the time I have real need for it.

For the moment, however, Ross's advice to people like me jibes with my decision earlier this month: "If you're getting by with your current aid, hold on for a little while longer. The digital revolution, and a whole generation of new aids, is just around the corner."

A New Member 3 OCTOBER 1997

Welcome to the club. This morning's papers report that President Clinton is getting two unobtrusive in-the-ear-canal aids to compensate for his loss of high-frequency hearing. We can empathize, Mr. President . . . all twenty-eight million of us Americans who, the National Institutes of Health report (according to this morning's *New York Times*), now live with hearing loss or deafness, but especially the five million of us who use assistive devices.

The president's loss is of the typical high-frequency variety and, given his relative youth, is attributed to too much rock music and rifle fire during his early years. Noise-induced hearing loss tends to occur at high frequencies. (In the aging ear, such loss is called presbycusis.) The papers report that he plans to wear the aids only in crowd situations, where hearing is especially challenging.

Note: he *plans* to wear them. His doctors have recommended them, and he *says* he will wear them. Mr. President, many of us five million predict that you won't initially, before adapting, find these an unmitigated blessing. Moreover, you sometimes will "forget" to, or decide not to, use them. Bear with the distraction of your own altered voice and the amplified extraneous sounds. You *will* hear better. And perhaps you, as a fifty-two-year-old, will be able to do what the older President Reagan (a fellow hearing-aid wearer) could not: help encourage hearing-aid use, when needed, by younger or middle-aged people.

Words that Hurt 10 NOVEMBER 1997

"Never mind." How familiar those words are to the hard of hearing.

"Ted said that the doctor wanted her . . ."

"I'm sorry?"

"Ted said that the doctor wanted her . . ."

"Ted said what?"

"Oh, never mind."

Sometimes the information is trivial and not worth the effort of repetition. Sometimes the words are spoken for my ears only, and so cannot be spoken more loudly.

Regardless, "never mind" is an acknowledgment of mutual frustration and failure. With these words—among the easiest to lip-read because of their context and familiarity—typically comes a brief flash of pain: a reminder of your deficiency, a twinge of loss, a fleeting awareness that you will never know what it was that, an instant ago, seemed worth saying.

I do not blame those who utter those stinging words, which sometimes are accompanied by a shake of the head, rolled eyes, or a dismissive gesture. What else should people do? What would I do in their place? Still, I am grateful that my sensitive and clear-voiced closest friends—is their clear articulation one reason they are my closest friends?—never utter those words. At least not yet.

A Loving Partner to the End 18 NOVEMBER 1997

For seven decades my father and mother have been an oasis for each other. They met while riding a commuter ferry from Seattle to Bainbridge Island, fell in love, and married only after saving money to pay off debts. With an aunt's assistance, they built their first home, without indoor plumbing, for $1,012. After nearly twenty years of marriage, about the time my memories of them began, they still were joyfully in love. Each day as Dad returned home, they greeted each other with a warm embrace and the sort of kiss that said, "I love you." She was a dedicated mother of four, a skilled homemaker, and a gracious hostess at many dinners and parties in our home. She was also utterly loyal to Dad. When he was out of earshot, she often reminded us children how hard he worked and how honorable he was. To her, he was a great man, as he is to his children.

In her later years, as silence encroached on her world, he became her helpmeet and safe haven. Much as he would have liked to socialize with friends and travel, he never strayed far from her side. He translated for her using their pidgin signs, with his familiar lips slowly forming words, and especially using their writing boards. As she grew weaker, he dressed her, bathed her, assisted her in the bathroom, and at night helped her get ready for bed. "She was there for me for so many years. Now it is my time to be there for her." Aware of her dependence on him—someone else could take over the nursing care, but no one could replace his companionship—all of us wished that in the end she would not be left alone.

Last week, that wish was granted. Dad, still able-bodied and clear of mind at eighty-nine, was with her when the sweet chariot swung low to carry her home. In her final days, however, even he could not reach her. When she was moaning in pain during her brief waking periods, struggling to communicate, not even he could make out her indistinct words. Her isolation was now complete.

As an extended family held together by the faith of our parents, we like to imagine that "great gettin'-up morning" when, in the vision of John of Patmos, God "will wipe away every tear from their eyes. Death shall be no more; mourning and crying and pain will be no more, for the first things have passed away," and all things are made new. In my vision of this hoped-for reality, the ears of the deaf once again hear a bird's song, a friend's intimate words, a lover's approach . . . and Mother leaps up to embrace her life partner and to laugh again.

Back in real time, I wonder whether I will be called on to provide similar support for Carol later in life (or she for me). If I am, I cannot be sure that I will be capable of Dad's patient, gentle, self-sacrificing love. But this much I know. I know whom I will remember.

When Not Hearing Seems Like Not Caring 6 FEBRUARY 1998

As Laura and I finished our weekly lunch date this afternoon, a stranger approached, asking, "Are you David Myers?" When I indicated that I was, he said, speaking slowly, "I want to thank you." "You're welcome," I replied with a silly grin. But then, in a low voice that I couldn't make out, he explained something further. I gathered that he was thanking me for my book on happiness, which had meant a lot to him, and for an ABC television special in which I had played a part. I thanked him more genuinely for his kind words, and he walked off with a friend.

"That wasn't very sensitive," Laura then observed.

"What did he say?" I inquired. "He said he was a grieving father—his daughter died last month." Oh dear, I think remorsefully, able in light of this information to replay his telling me that his daughter, Carla, had died. I had missed the "grieving father" statement and was trying to recollect whether I had known his daughter. On a scale of 1 to 10, my ability to empathize must have registered at about 1. (Later I recalled that his daughter had been the victim of a local traffic accident, and I wrote him a note of condolence.) On how many other occasions, without

Laura there to brief me, have I unknowingly bungled a sensitive situation?

Comparisons

24 APRIL 1998

Ten days ago, I thought I'd lost the hearing in my left ear. For several days it had seemed plugged, as if by water. When I visited my physician, he needed only a two-second peek into the ear canal: "You've got a middle-ear infection."

Five days on antibiotics brought no change. Now that the hearing aid was useless, meetings and group conversation slid below my auditory threshold. From the infection (and perhaps the antibiotics and minimal auditory input also played a role) tinnitus—ringing in the ear—began to set in. Tinnitus is to someone who is hard of hearing what sensations of a phantom limb are to an amputee, or visual hallucinations to someone after prolonged sensory deprivation. After an ear infection or sensory deprivation, the pertinent brain areas seem to manufacture their own activity, often experienced as a steady tone.

Finally, after a week, the infection has cleared up and my hearing has returned. The payback is that I now for the time being feel grateful to be better off than I was. It is often so in life. Our emotions depend on our comparisons. The tent floor underneath the sleeping bag makes the bed back home feel softer. The Lenten bowls of rice make the roast chicken afterward tastier. After temporary separation from a loved one, the reunion is sweet, the person less taken for granted. Indeed, there is no better way to reframe our thinking, our attitude, our gratitude, than to experience reminders of our blessings.

The experience of having one ear plugged also, however, gave me a glimpse of what might lay ahead. And it triggered this thought: During disability awareness week on campus, students simulate paralysis by going about in wheelchairs. They simulate blindness by wearing blindfolds. Why not also outfit some of these empathy-seeking students with earplugs that simulate hearing loss? "I have often thought it would be a blessing if each human being were stricken blind and deaf for a few days during his early adult life," wrote Helen Keller. "Darkness would make him more appreciative of sight; silence would teach him the joys of sound."

Advice for Friends and Family Members 15 MAY 1998

New books for the hard of hearing by Anne Pope (*Hear*) and Marcia Dugan (*Keys to Living with Hearing Loss*) offer excellent tips for their friends, colleagues, and family members. Would you like us to understand you? Take these hints:

Invite us to a quiet place—a carpeted restaurant or one with booths, a room without music blaring, a chair away from the air conditioning.

Get our attention. If we're reading or watching television, make sure we are looking at you.

Face the light and face us. It helps us to see your mouth (we all do some lipreading). So take the pencil or gum out, keep your hands away from your face, and (if you're a hard-to-hear bearded husband) consider shaving. Don't think us rude if we watch your mouth instead of your eyes.

Rephrase. If we don't get it, restate it. Lipreading helps us (as will videophones), but only about one-third of speech is visible on the lips. *Tight* and *fight* will not be confused (feel your lips speaking them). *Thrash* can be lip-read, because the consonant phonemes (*th*, *r*, and *sh*) are all visibly formed by the lips and teeth (go look in the mirror). But *got* and *cot* look the same, because the difference is formed in the back of the throat. *Sip* and *zip* also look the same, as do *toe* and *doe*—because *s*, *z*, *t*, and *d* are formed by the tongue inside the mouth. *Pat*, *mat*, and *bat*, too, look the same on the lips, though not on the invisible tongue. So try using different words to express the same concept. Restate "Do you want anything from the store?" as "Can I get you something at Safeway?" (Fortunately, understanding consists of more than lipreading, because nonverbal communication helps—your gestures, frowns, and intensities help us discern your meaning.)

Create a context. Give us a clue what the subject is. Have a printed agenda for the meeting, or use visual aids. Caller I.D. is a godsend for the hard of hearing. (Lacking context and clues, we may otherwise struggle to catch the caller's identity.)

Speak slowly. Don't shout, but do help our brains to accomplish what computers have such great difficulty doing with human voice—break down the stream of speech sounds into individual words. Remember how an unfamiliar language sounds to you: the words all seem to run together. Speak each word distinctly, with pauses between phrases and sentences. As many a grandparent has advised, "slow down and enunciate more clearly!"

TABLE 5.1 Self Help for Hard of Hearing People's Tips for . . .

Hearing People on Communicating with Hard of Hearing People	**Hard of Hearing People on Communicating with Hearing People**
• Set Your Stage: Face audience directly. Spotlight your face. Avoid noisy backgrounds. Get attention first. Ask how you can help communicate.	• Set Your Stage: Tell others how best to talk to you. Pick your best spot (light, quiet, proximity). Anticipate difficult situations, plan how to minimize them.
• Project Your Communication: Don't shout. Speak clearly, at a moderate pace. Don't hide your mouth, chew food or gum, or smoke while talking. Rephrase if you are not understood. Use facial expressions, gestures. Give clues when changing subject.	• Project Your Communication: Pay attention. Concentrate on speaker. Look for visual clues. Ask for written cues if needed. Don't interrupt. Let conversation flow awhile to gain more meaning.
• Establish Empathy with Audience: Be patient if response seems slow. Stay positive and relaxed. Talk *to* a hard of hearing person, not about him or her. Offer respect to help build confidence.	• Establish Empathy with Audience: React. Let speaker know how well he is doing. Don't bluff. Admit when you don't understand. If too tired to concentrate, ask for discussion later.

Ask us if we have heard. Remember, we hate to seem inept and to embarrass both of us by volunteering that we could not hear.

Self Help for Hard of Hearing People provides further tips (Table 5.1).

Audiologist-writer Mark Ross encourages those of us with hearing loss to ask people to do these things—to practice "assertive listening." When eating out with friends, we should tell them that we'd prefer a place that's not noisy. Explain to the person taking the reservation or seating us: "I have a hearing loss, and it would help me if we could be seated in a quiet corner." Explain to the server, "I don't hear well. It would help me if you could turn the music down a little." Choose a seat in the corner. Ask conversational partners to "say that again, more slowly" (in which case they will also articulate more carefully). Seek clarification about exactly what you missed ("What did you say her name was?"). In conversation, minimize "speaker-to-listener distance." (With distance from a speaker, the signal [voice]-to-noise ratio plummets.) At events, sit front and center. Arrange the living room furniture in a tight circle. Meet around the smallest possible table.

A Noisy World 16 MAY 1998

"Invite us to a quiet place." If only there were more quiet places. Many restaurants, it seems to me, are designed by architects who bear a grudge against the hard of hearing (or, more likely, don't even think of them). They use hard surfaces that reflect sound to help create a sense of energy (or for some of us stress). The music blares. To be heard above the noise, people raise their voices, and the chaos is compounded.

Mark Ross reports that "the deleterious effect of noise upon speech comprehension is the most frequent complaint made by people with hearing loss." That's because hearing requires a good signal-to-noise ratio. In an acoustically unfriendly environment, conventional hearing aids don't solve the problem, because they amplify both signals and reverberating noise. (The new generation of digital aids aims to dampen restaurant or airplane noise while amplifying the voice you want to hear.) Thus I have long fantasized about helping launch a nationwide chain of tea rooms and coffee houses to be called The Quiet Place. With carpeted floors, acoustical ceilings, covered walls, and high booths, my Quiet Place franchises would offer people a cozy place for relaxed, intimate conversation, confidential meetings, and quiet reading. *Hearing Health* recently congratulated the *San Francisco Chronicle* for including decibel ratings in their restaurant reviews and rating noise at peak hours by showing between one bell (quietest) and four bells (almost 80 decibels), or a bomb for the very loudest.

The Quiet Places would also be busy, successful places, if one can believe the results of a survey appearing in the January 1998 issue of *Bon Appétit.* Forty-four percent of restaurant patrons reported that noise was their least favorite aspect of the dining experience. If restaurants were to offer noise-free as well as smoke-free areas—without loud music or hard, sound-reflecting surfaces—I'll wager that customers would seek them out.

Classrooms often suffer the same problem. Thankfully, the Acoustical Society of America (www.acoustics.org) has a task force devoted to classroom acoustics. Its goal is to "eliminate acoustical barriers to classroom learning, and to develop guidelines and standards for good acoustics in schools." Thinking of the classroom as a listening environment will help not only students with hearing losses but also young children and those who are struggling to learn and use a new language. These groups all require a higher signal-to-noise ratio than do the adult architects with normal hearing who design these spaces.

Just As I Am 28 MAY 1998

I have been granted a reprieve. Sensing that my hearing was hardly better with the hearing aid, I had the aid checked . . . and was delighted to receive it back with its volume restored to a level I haven't enjoyed in months. (An accumulation of ear wax was the problem, and a simple cleaning was the solution. Ear wax inhibits bacteria, repels insects, and cleans the ear, so I know I should love it. But sometimes it's a nuisance.)

Suddenly I am hearing all sorts of things I have been missing, and I am much less worried about the meeting I am about to enter. Never have I appreciated the once-disliked hearing aid so much.

My mild elation makes me empathize with Stephen Kuusisto, who writes in *Planet of the Blind* (1998) of his life journey into acknowledged blindness. Although Kuusisto was born premature and with limited vision, he and his parents resisted his taking on the identity of a blind person. Instead, "seeing through glasses darkly," he struggled to ride a bicycle, navigate independently, and attend regular school—all the while falling frequently, being unable to play sports or see a blackboard, and enduring endless taunts and humiliations. In Helsinki, "needing assistance and failing to disclose it, I must act more sighted, seem jaunty and independent. . . . but inwardly I'm in a swarm of sightless panic. . . . I'm addicted to appearing independent. Every step is a lie. Step, lie. Step, lie. My angels are giddy, just beyond the bounds of life, watching me."

Gradually, he comes to accept his disability. "Why should it take so long for me to like the blind self?" he muses, echoing the struggles that many who are hard of hearing experience in a similar way. "I resist it, admit it, then resist again, as though blindness were a fetish, a perverse weakness, a thing I could overcome with the force of will power." And then one day he takes the big step: "I call the telephone operator and ask for the number for the New York State Commission for the Blind. I need help walking. I've needed help all my life. It's that simple."

He begins to use a cane and discovers that not only does he fall less often but people—now that they understand—suddenly become more accepting and helpful. Not long after adopting the cane, Kuusisto graduates to a guide dog. The experience is exhilarating:

> For the first time I feel the sunken lanes under my feet.
>
> The street is more my own. I belong here.
>
> I'm walking without the fight-or-flee gunslinger crouch that has been the lifelong measure of blindness.
>
> I'm not frightened by the general onslaught of sensation.
>
> The harness is a transmitter, the dog is confident.
>
> At every curb we come to a reliable and firm stop. I cannot fall. . . .

> Faith moves from belief into conviction, then to certainty.
>
> We are a self-conferred powerhouse, we two.
>
> At age thirty-nine I learn to walk upright.
>
> With the help of classmates and the trainers, I am choosing to be blind in a forceful way. I even begin to enjoy my mistakes. . . .
>
> Why didn't I yield to this earlier? Why did I take so long?
>
> It doesn't matter, I'm doing it now. . . .
>
> Not everyone with vision loss goes through this long struggle with self-consciousness. There are those who lose their vision suddenly and find tremendous powers of resilience. They give hope to the people around them, both the sighted and the blind.
>
> We are, all of us, ecstatic creatures, capable of joyous mercy to the self and to others. . . . Sometimes roses grow on the sheer banks of the sea cliff.

Those on the gentler journey from sound to silence can understand Stephen Kuusisto's valiant effort not to appear impaired. After missing the punch line, we offer fraudulent laughter—a reflexive mimicry of those around us, our strategy for keeping our impairment invisible. But we also understand Kuusisto's relief at letting go of the illusion and finding help. Even in my simple delight at regaining an effective hearing aid I glimpse his ecstasy.

A Rich and Useful Language — 10 JUNE 1998

In the June 5 issue of the *Chronicle of Higher Education,* State University of New York at Binghamton professor Lennard Davis reflects on the recent controversial vote of the University of Virginia faculty "to allow American Sign

Language to fulfill the foreign-language requirement for an undergraduate degree." As a child of deaf parents who learned American Sign Language before learning English, he understands that ASL's complex dance of fingers, hands, face, and body is a rich language that is definitely foreign to English. Moreover, he notes, "the utility of learning sign language goes beyond the ability to speak with the deaf. The fact is, a person is far more likely to become deaf than, for example, to become French. As many baby boomers, from President Clinton on down, begin to lose their hearing and rely on hearing aids, it seems logical that more people should learn sign language. How many elderly, hard-of-hearing members of the family, struggling with their hearing aids at the dinner table, left out of the conversation, could be accommodated if they and their families had had the foresight to learn sign language." And why not? With no disrespect intended to French-speakers or to those who taught me French in high school and college so that I could meet certain language requirements and pass a graduate school language exam, I wish now that I could have studied sign language instead. Except for a few days in Paris and Montreal, I have made no conscious use of my limited French. A basic knowledge of signing, gained at an age when the facility for such learning is greater, would be likelier to prove useful eventually (and to give insight into the mindset and culture of the deaf).

Pratfalls — 15 AUGUST 1998

Recent issues of *Hearing Health* offer more examples of the pratfalls of the hard of hearing. Editor Paula Bonillas gave her daughter castanets for Christmas . . . when really she had wished for a *casting net*. One reader recalled asking for her husband at a YMCA desk. Not understanding the clerk who asked her to "please wait here," she followed him . . . and ended up standing before a naked man in the men's locker room. As another reader, driving on a rainy night, pulled into a 7–Eleven parking lot, she heard her companions yell "Go!" and rammed into a passing car. (They actually had yelled "No!")

6

Understanding Hearing and Its Loss

Testing, Testing 21 OCTOBER 1998

I revisited my audiologist today to have a retest and discuss the emerging digital hearing-aid technology. Both ears have worsened a bit, and the hearing in my "good" right ear, he told me afterward, is now what it was in my "bad" left ear several years ago. I infer that I am still following Mother's lead. The doctor and I agree that I will be a customer for a new digital aid that becomes available in early 1999.

The tests given by my audiologist fascinate me. The audiogram (Figure 6.1) illustrates the data generated by a typical testing session. You listen to a descending series of pure tones at each of several frequency levels. The audiologist's instruction is simple: When you hear a tone, press the hand-held button. My responses often feel somewhat arbitrary—did I just hear a tone, or was I imagining it? Yet across testings the audiological exam is remarkably reliable at determining the threshold for hearing at different frequencies in each ear.

Figure 6.1 My Audiogram

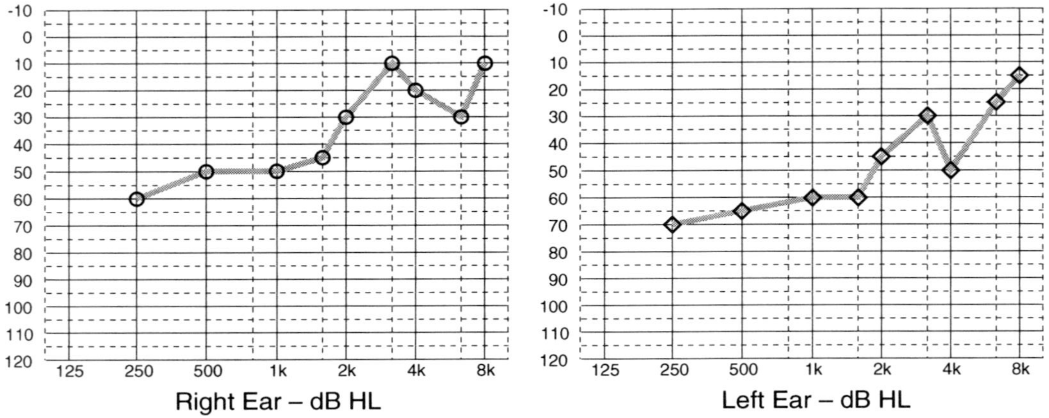

Familiar images come to mind as I study the audiogram. Hitting a piano key triggers a sound wave, which is nothing more than jostling molecules of air, each bumping into the next, as a shove is transmitted through a stadium's crowded exit tunnel. It's also like water ripples circling out from where a tossed stone has broken the surface of a pond. As we swim in our ocean of moving air molecules, our ears detect brief air pressure changes. They then transform them into nerve impulses, which our brain decodes as sounds.

The strength or intensity of these waves of molecules as they strike our eardrums determines their loudness, measured in decibels. The softest sound humans normally hear is designated as 0 decibels. Every 10 decibels corresponds to a tenfold increase. Normal conversation (60 decibels) is a thousand times louder than a 30-decibel whisper. And a passing subway train (100 decibels) is *ten billion* times more intense than the faintest detectable sound! Our sensitivity to both extremely faint and extremely intense sounds, from rustling leaves to a cracking limb, was surely a boon to survival when our ancestors were hunting or being hunted.

A University of Illinois web page on audiology further explains our "amazing" sensitivity. An erg is the energy required to lift a milligram (one-thousandth of a gram) a quarter of an inch. That's not much energy. Yet most humans can detect as sound an air pressure disturbance that represents a mere billionth of an erg. If our ears were much more sensitive, we would hear a constant hiss from the random movements of air molecules.

Sound waves also vary in frequency, from the long, slow waves produced by distant thunder to the short, fast waves of the high-pitched piccolo. A healthy young adult's ear picks up a remarkable range of wave frequencies, from those arriving at 20 cycles per second to those at 20,000 cycles per second. The human ear hears best those sounds with frequencies of 500 to 8,000 hertz, a range that—wonder of wonders—just happens to correspond to the range of the human voice.

Human words, however, are complex sounds, offering a mix of frequencies. Vowel sounds are mostly lower-frequency. Consonant sounds (such as *d*, *t*, and *s*, though not *m* and *n*) are higher-frequency. Most age-related decline in hearing is for higher-frequency sounds, as revealed in the downward-sloping line of an audiogram. When the high-frequency consonant sounds become less audible while lower-frequency background noise still comes in clear, it becomes difficult to distinguish speech against background noise.[1]

My unusual "reverse-slope" hearing loss, however, is greatest for low-frequency sounds. (Impaired though I may be, I challenge any reader of this book to a hearing contest only for faint 3,000-hertz sounds directed to the right ear.) No matter how much trouble I may have with owls and vowels, my hearing is still adequate for most consonant sounds. I guess I should count myself fortunate, because consonants carry more information than vowels. The treth ef thes stetement shed be evedent frem thes bref demonstretien. For human speech, the consonant-laden 3,000- to 6,000-hertz range is critical.

After an audiogram assesses the extent of hearing loss

1. For an effective simulation of typical hearing loss—how speech sounds with the higher frequencies muted—visit www.neurophys.wisc.edu/animations.

in decibels, an audiologist may draw on a descriptive table that classifies the loss. The audiologist finds that the audiograms for my ears show a hearing loss that is moderate (in the right ear) to moderately severe (in the left ear)—but only for low frequencies (Table 6.1). That explains why I experience the most difficulty in hearing people with soft, low (often male) voices.

If a person is profoundly impaired at particular frequencies—functionally deaf—then amplifying sound at those frequencies simply won't help. That's where "frequency-transposition hearing aids" may someday enter the picture. For most people, this will mean *lowering* the frequency output. The latest devices, reports Mark Ross (in *Hearing Loss,* May–June 1998), don't just lower high-pitched sounds to lower-pitched sounds (or the reverse for people like me). They lower the output *proportionally.*

TABLE 6.1

Loss	*Classification*	*Effects*
0 to 15 decibels	Normal hearing	
16 to 25 decibels	Slight hearing loss	Slight difficulty with soft speech
25 to 40 decibels	Mild hearing loss	Difficulty with soft speech
41 to 55 decibels	Moderate hearing loss	Frequent difficulty with normal speech
56 to 70 decibels	Moderately severe loss	Occasional difficulty with loud speech
71 to 90 decibels	Severe hearing loss	Frequent difficulty with loud speech
over 90 decibels	Profound hearing loss	Near total loss of hearing

If 8,000 hertz input is lowered to 4,000 hertz, and 4,000 hertz input is lowered to 2,000 hertz, then women's voices will still be higher than men's, and "a woman would still sound like a woman and not like a male baritone with a frog in his throat."

The Wonder of It All 28 DECEMBER 1998

The more I contemplate the universe, life, and the human senses, the more awestruck I am. The odds that the universe would be born with just the right amount of matter and force so that it neither collapses back in on itself nor explodes into a soup too thin for stars, and that intelligent life would then form, are so infinitesimal that they evoke a spiritual sense of wonder. (The universe more and more seems so improbably yet precisely welcoming toward us as to lend renewed credibility to the idea of a providential First Cause, "to which everyone gives the name of God," as Aquinas said.)

Those susceptible to being wonderstruck, however, need look no further than human sensation. "The larger the island of knowledge," noted the preacher Ralph Sockman, "the longer the shoreline of wonder." Indeed, the more I learn about sensation, the more convinced I am that what is truly extraordinary is not *extra*sensory perception (claims for which have time and again dissolved under close scrutiny) but rather our very ordinary moment-to-moment organizing of formless neural impulses into colorful sights and meaningful sounds. Sherlock Holmes had it right (in *A Study in Scarlet*): "The most commonplace crime is often the most mysterious. . . .

Life is infinitely stranger than anything which the mind of man could invent. We would not dare to conceive the things which are really mere commonplaces of existence."

Vision gets the most attention, and justifiably so. A huge area of the brain is devoted to vision—ten times as much as to hearing. As we are reading a sentence like this, something amazing is happening. Particles of light energy are being absorbed by the receptor cells of our eyes and are then converted into neural signals. These signals activate neighboring cells, which process the information for a third layer of cells; they converge to form a nerve tract that transmits a million electrochemical messages per moment up to the brain. The brain divides a visual scene into subdimensions such as color, depth, movement, and form and works on each aspect simultaneously. Finally, in some mysterious way, it assembles the component features into a consciously perceived image, which is instantly compared with previously stored images and recognized as words we know.

The whole process is rather like taking apart a house, splinter by splinter, transporting it to a different location, and then, through the work of millions of specialized workers, putting it back together. What is more, all of this takes place in a fraction of a second. The more I explore ordinary sensation, the more I empathize with Job: "I have uttered what I did not understand, things too wonderful for me."

But I can't dismiss hearing as the poor sister of sight—or as what some researchers have called the Cinderella sense. I've been reading a new book, *From Sound to Synapse: Physiology of the Mammalian Ear* (1998), by retired University of Wisconsin neurophysiologist C. Daniel Geisler. Geisler suggests that anyone who will consider the "astonishing and elegant mechanisms" by which we hear "will come to share my great sense of awe for this beautiful system."

Here, in a snapshot, is the delicate process by which we transform sound pressure waves into our experience of hearing. The points where it might go awry show up clearly, too, and help me understand my own condition (Figure 6.2).

The process involves an intricate conversion of sound waves to other wave forms: the visible outer ear collects the sound waves and channels them to the eardrum. If wax buildup, a cyst, or some object blocks the ear canal, the ability to hear diminishes. The odd shape of the outer ear helps us distinguish sounds from above and below. An 11 September 1998 *Science* article reports that when Dutch researchers fitted people with plastic ears with altered

Figure 6.2 How Sound Travels from Ear to Brain

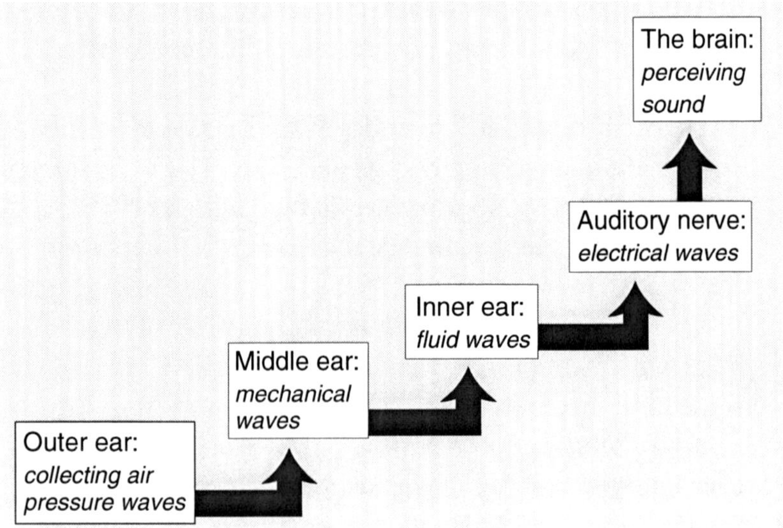

ridges it "completely disrupted perceptions of whether sounds were coming from above or below."

The eardrum's vibrations transmit the sound waves through the three tiny bones of the middle ear—the hammer, anvil, and stirrup (Figure 6.3). If ear infections or damage to one of these bones interferes with mechanical conduction, a person will suffer "conductive hearing loss." (That was my problem during last April's ear infection, which probably caused a buildup of fluid behind the eardrum.) A middle-ear conduction problem can sometimes also be resolved by ear surgery. If middle-ear conduction is nonexistent, a hearing instrument that transmits sound through the skull can provide partial, muffled hearing. (The audiologist's test for loss of middle-ear conduction always amazes me: it is possible to *hear* vibrations via the skull!)

These relayed vibrations strike a membrane covering the beginning of cochlea, the inner ear's snail-shaped, fluid-filled tube. The vibrations initiate a fluid pressure wave, causing ripples on the cochlea's basilar membrane, which is lined with tiny hairlike projections called hair cells. As the basilar membrane ripples, the hair cells bend, rather like a wheat field bending in the wind. Their bending triggers impulses in the adjacent nerve fibers that converge to form the auditory nerve up to the brain.

Curiously, 80 percent of the nerves from each ear connect to the temporal lobe on the opposite side of the brain. Even a phantom ringing sound, if heard in the right ear, is associated with activity in the *left* temporal lobe. This pretty much mirrors the body's cross-wiring for touch sensations and muscle control. A stroke that immobilizes the left leg has damaged the right hemisphere.

Figure 6.3 The Hearing Mechanism

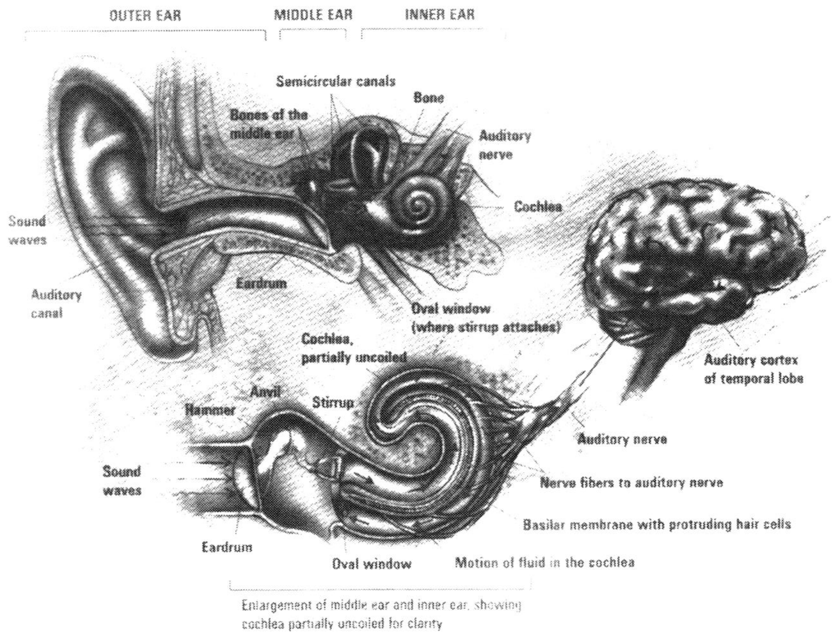

Source: David G. Myers, *Psychology,* 5th ed. Used by permission of Worth Publishers.

Common sensorineural hearing loss—my own affliction and that of more than nine in ten older adults who lose hearing—results from damaged hair cells or loss of nerve fibers leading from the cochlea (which reminds me of the squirrels nibbling on our phone lines). The proportion of each is difficult to distinguish clinically; thus "sensorineural" is more apt a term than "nerve deafness." For deaf children, the culprit may sometimes have been rubella or syphilis in the mother during pregnancy, oxygen deprivation after birth, or meningitis. For adults who lose hearing, Ménière's disease is sometimes to blame (an inner-ear disorder that can disrupt balance and cause nausea, hearing loss, and ringing in the ears). Sometimes it is drugs (aminoglycoside antibiotics such as streptomycin). But more often it is genetically influenced atrophy, or—for a reported one-third of people with hearing loss—toxic noise. So it is not surprising that hearing, like the other senses, declines with age (Figures 6.4 and 6.5). A 1997 report of the National Center for Health Statistics revealed that 71 percent of America's 4.2 million noninstitutionalized hearing-aid wearers were sixty-five or older.

From vibrating air to moving piston to fluid waves to electrical impulses to the brain: we hear. The system's speed, accuracy, and intricacy is astounding. Its intricacy is especially breathtaking when viewed close at hand. The most magical element in the process is the hair cells, damage to which accounts for most hearing loss. (For frequencies at which there has been more than an 80-decibel loss, the relevant hair cells are so far gone that amplification at that frequency does little good.)

A Howard Hughes Medical Institute report on these "quivering bundles that let us hear" remarks on their "extreme sensitivity and extreme speed." A cochlea only has sixteen thousand of them, says the Hughes report, some three-fourths of which are outer hair cells, the rest the supersensitive inner hair cells. (The inner hair cells have several phone lines—nerve fibers—coming into each of their homes; the outer cells, which help amplify the incoming signals, share party lines.)

Sixteen thousand cells sounds like a lot until we compare them with the 100 million or so photoreceptors in the eye. But the inner hair cells are extraordinarily responsive. If the tiny bundles of cilia on the tip of a hair cell are deflected by merely the width of an atom—the equivalent of displacing the top of the Eiffel Tower by only half an inch—the alert hair cell triggers a neural response. Moreover, at the highest perceived frequency they can turn neural current on and off 20 thousand times per sec-

Figure 6.4 Percentage of Americans with Hearing Loss (26 dB or Greater)

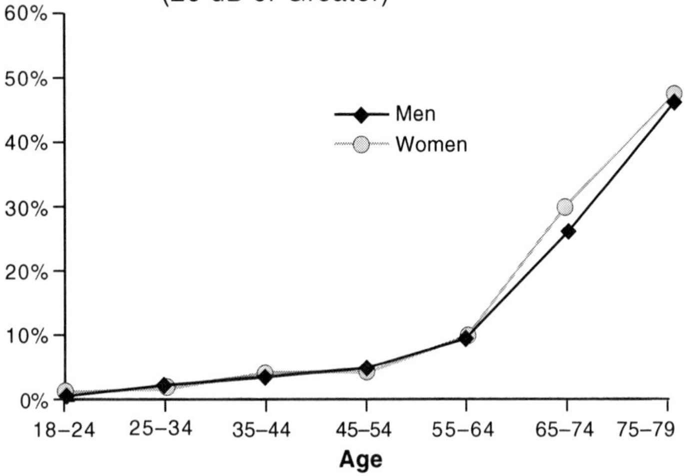

Source: National Center for Health Statistics, 1960–62.

Figure 6.5 Percentage of Americans Who Cannot Hear and Understand Normal Speech, by Age

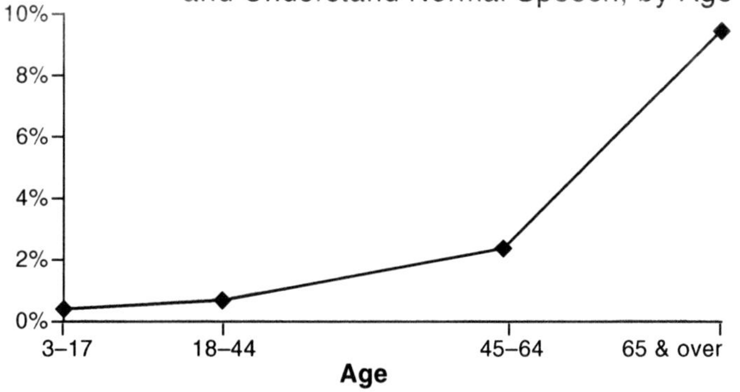

Source: National Health Survey of 93,327 households, reported in *Prevalence and Characteristics of Persons with Hearing Trouble: United States, 1990-1991. Vital and Health Statistics*, series 10, no. 188, March 1994.

ond! As you might expect of something so sensitive, however, they are delicate and fragile. Blast them with incessant noise from a jackhammer or headset and the cilia will begin to wither or fuse. Although rock and roll may be here to stay, the sad truth for some rock musicians is that their hearing—and that of their listeners—may not be.

How do we detect loudness? It's not, as one might suppose, from the intensity of a hair cell's response. A soft, pure tone activates only the few hair cells attuned to its frequency. If the sound is louder, the neighboring hair cells also respond. Thus, the brain interprets loudness by the number of hair cells activated.

If a hair cell loses sensitivity to soft sounds, it may still respond to loud sounds. This helps explain another surprise: really loud sounds may seem equally loud to people with and without hearing loss. On hearing loud music, I have often wondered how much louder it must sound to people with normal hearing. I now understand that it probably sounds much to them as it does to me. This is why people with hearing impairments don't want *all* sounds (loud and soft) amplified, as happens with traditional hearing aids. We like sound *compressed*—which means that soft sounds are amplified more than loud ones. By minimally amplifying potentially damaging loud noises, sound compression helps protect our ears.

Brain Power — 29 DECEMBER 1998

We say that we hear with our ears, but it would be more exact to say that we hear with our brain. My brain, not my ears, allows me to pick up the phone and instantly recognize a friend's voice among the thousands of voices I have heard. Three other phenomena further demonstrate hearing to be a phenomenon of our active brain.

Tinnitus. If a tree does *not* fall in the forest but someone hears it, is it a sound? So far as the brain is concerned it certainly is, notes University of Connecticut psychologist David Miller. At one time or another some four in five people with sensorineural hearing loss hear sounds, usually steady tones, that are not there. Even surgically destroying the inner ear does not guarantee an end to this tinnitus, which must therefore, like an amputee's phantom-limb sensations, be the creation of the brain. The same is true of the phantom smells and tastes that some people experience following nerve damage. There is more to perception than meets the senses!

A recent report in the *Proceedings of the National Academy of Sciences* by a German research team led by Werner Muhlnickel pinpoints brain activity during tinnitus. Earlier brain scans had shown that the auditory cortex, the area in the brain that processes sound, is active when schizophrenia patients experience auditory hallucinations. This new research similarly situates the source of tinnitus.

The cochlea's sound receptors for differing frequencies connect to corresponding frequency locations in the brain. The brain areas that respond to tones of, say, 1,000, 2,000, 3,000, 4,000, and 5,000 hertz are located along a fairly straight line. Pipe a 4,000-hertz tone into the ear, and the brain becomes active at its spot for receiving 4,000-hertz input. But when a tinnitus patient hears a phantom 4,000-hertz tone, the brain becomes active several millimeters away from the normal location for 4,000-hertz reception. A similar shift in brain activity away from the expected position occurs with amputees experiencing sensations in a phantom limb. In both cases, the loss of input seems to alter the brain. And in both cases the brain is creating its own vivid sensory experiences.

Locating sounds. Another example of the wonders of hearing is how the brain computes a sound's location (Figure 6.6). Why don't we have just one big ear—perhaps in our forehead above our nose?

For a couple of reasons, two ears are better than one. If a bell rings on your right, your right ear receives a more intense sound slightly sooner than your left ear. Because sound travels 750 miles per hour and our ears are but six inches apart, the difference in loudness and the time lag are not great. A "just noticeable difference" in the direction from which two sounds come corresponds to a time difference of just 0.000027 seconds. But our brain can detect such infinitesimal differences, and it uses them to locate the sound. An owl's brain (and probably a human's, too) processes time differences in one area of the brain and differences in intensity in another, before the information on both is merged to pinpoint where the sound is coming from.

When a sound comes from a spot equidistant from our two ears (directly ahead, behind, overhead, or beneath us), locating the sound becomes trickier. Thanks to the shape of our outer ear, we are able to glean some indication, but we can gather no added clues from differences in timing and intensity. When we mislocate a sound, it is usually coming from within this zone in which the two ears are receiving identical input. Here is a demonstration that

Figure 6.6 Locating Sound

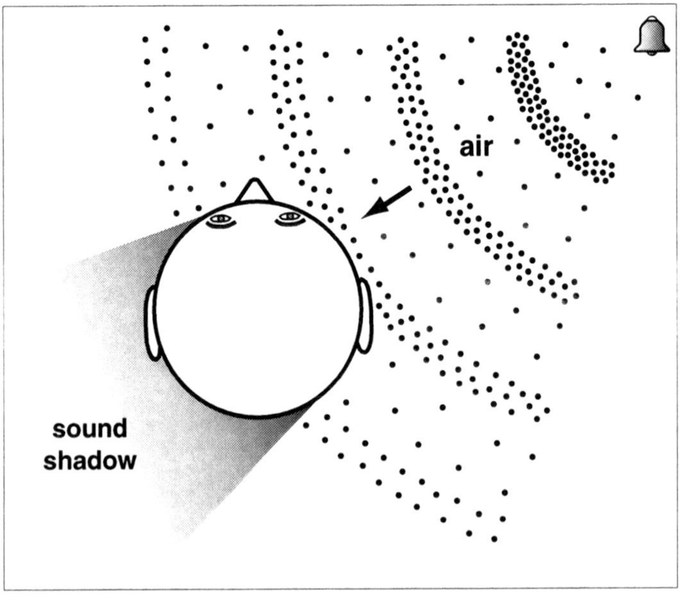

Source: *From Sound to Synapse: The Physiology of the Mammalian Ear*, by C. Daniel Geisler. Copyright © 1998 by C. Daniel Geisler. Used by permission of Oxford University Press.

anyone can try at home. While a student sits with eyes closed, I snap my fingers or click a clicker at various locations around the head. The student easily points to the sound when it comes from either side but is more hesitant and prone to error when it comes from ahead, behind, above, or below.

Perceptual set. In a C-SPAN lecture yesterday evening, Bill Gates mentioned that the Microsoft team working on speech recognition calls itself the Wreck a Nice Beach Group—because their task is to enable computers to detect the difference between that phrase and the acoustically similar "recognize speech." The brain excels at such tasks. If someone says "I scream, you scream, we all scream for ice cream," we instantly and effortlessly hear the words as written here. To our ears, those screams are all the same, but not to the interpreting brain.

Experiments in cases where the two hemispheres of the brain have been surgically separated (to control epilepsy) demonstrate the speed and ease with which the brain performs interpretations. The verbal, left hemisphere, which acts as the brain's press agent, will do mental gymnastics to rationalize reactions it does not understand. If a patient follows an order sent to the right hemisphere ("Walk"), the left hemisphere will offer a ready explanation ("I'm going into the house to get a Coke"). Researcher Michael Gazzaniga concludes that the left hemisphere is an "interpreter" that instantly constructs theories to explain our behavior.

With equal speed, the interpreting brain fills in the gaps in our hearing. If it can make a plausible guess, it does. On asking, "What is that we just passed?" Gallaudet professor Samuel Trychin recalls hearing his companion in the car reply "Not very far." Believing that she had misunderstood, he repeated the question, only to hear again "Not very far"—rather than what she had actually said, "Knott's Berry Farm." Of course, people who are not hard of hearing miss or misperceive words, nursery rhymes, and song lyrics. One web site (www.kissthisguy.com) offers some 2,000 examples of such misperceptions.

How does the brain make these split-second guesses? As every psychology student learns, our experiences, assumptions, and expectations give us a perceptual set, or mental predisposition, that greatly influences what we perceive. The most familiar examples are visual. What we see in an ambiguous drawing or photo depends on what we are led to expect. On first viewing the "canals" on Mars through telescopes, some astronomers and writers perceived them to be the product of intelligent life. They were—but the intelligence was on the viewing end of the telescope.

Perceptual set also affects what we hear. Witness the kindly airline pilot who, on a takeoff run, looked over at his depressed copilot and said, "Cheer up." The copilot heard the usual "Gear up" and promptly raised the wheels—before they had left the ground.

When listening to rock music played backward, people often perceive an evil message *if* they are specifically told what to listen for. Again, this makes for a great class demonstration. The backward lyrics are gibberish on first hearing, but when they are replayed after students have been told what to expect, the class dissolves in laughter as everyone hears the ostensible message. In fact, it now becomes impossible *not* to hear those words.

The context in which words appear helps create our perceptual set. Did the critic advocate "attacks" on our politicians, or "a tax"? We must discern the meaning from the surrounding words. If it is clear that our conversational partner is talking about a restaurant, it becomes much easier to hear the words *menu* or *chef.*

One task of speech-recognition software will be to analyze the context and then retroactively impute meaning—something our brains do effortlessly. Imagine hearing a noise interrupted by the words "eel is on the wagon." Probably, we would instead perceive—we would actually hear—the first word as *wheel.* Given "eel is on the orange," we would hear *peel.* This curious phenomenon, discovered by Richard Warren, shows how the brain can work backward in time to allow a later stimulus to determine how we perceive an earlier one.

Selective attention. The best device for selectively amplifying the speech we want to hear above the surrounding noise remains the human brain. At any moment our brains focus our awareness on only a limited aspect of all that we are capable of experiencing. Until someone points it out, we've been unaware that our shoes are pressing against our feet or that our nose is in our line of vision. Now, suddenly, after these facts have been pointed out, the spotlight of our attention shifts, and our feet feel encased, while our nose stubbornly intrudes on the page before us.

Another example of the phenomenon of selective attention is the cocktail party effect—the ability to attend selectively to just one voice among many. Imagine hearing two conversations over a headset, one in each ear, and being asked to repeat the left-ear message as it is spoken.

When we pay attention to what is being said into the left ear, we don't perceive what is said into the right ear. If we are asked later what language the right ear heard, we may draw a blank (though we could recall the speaker's gender and loudness). At the level of conscious awareness, our attention is pretty much undivided.

So, yes, we hear with our brains, our amazing brains. The psalmist spoke more truth than he could have realized: "I am fearfully and wonderfully made."

A Time for Decisions — 1 JANUARY 1999

New Year's, a day for resolutions. At the beginning of this new year, I'm thinking about new beginnings that might be experienced by those of us who have become aware of hearing loss. It's a day when some of us ask ourselves, Do I need a hearing aid? Could I benefit from a newer one? If we are asking such questions, and if family members have been volunteering that I need one, the answer is likely to be Yes. Probably both I and they are having communication problems. It may be my hearing loss, but it's *our* problem.

We may initially have noticed the problem only occasionally—with certain people and in certain contexts. We do just fine, thank you, when people have the right vocal pitch, a familiar accent, clear articulation, good lip movement (with no beard), and moderately paced speech, especially in quiet settings or those with noise-absorbing acoustics. Yet we sometimes find ourselves cupping an ear or straining to hear someone. On entering the television room, a family member says for the umpteenth time,

"You've got that up awfully loud." In groups, we find ourselves pretending that we've heard, not wanting to become a real pain by asking people to repeat themselves every time we just don't get it. We may also talk too loud, as people naturally do when wearing a headset that disrupts their hearing.

So at what point do we need to consult an otolaryngologist (a physician specializing in the ear, nose, and throat), an audiologist (a professionally educated hearing specialist), or a center that dispenses hearing aids? The National Institute on Deafness and Other Communication Disorders (www.nih.gov/nidcd) has ten simple questions for us to answer (yes or no):

> Do you have a problem hearing over the telephone?
> Do you have trouble following the conversation when two or more people are talking at the same time?
> Do people complain that you turn the television volume up too high?
> Do you have to strain to understand conversation?
> Do you have trouble hearing in a noisy background?
> Do you find yourself asking people to repeat themselves?
> Do many people you talk to seem to mumble (or not speak clearly)?
> Do you misunderstand what others are saying and respond inappropriately?
> Do you have trouble understanding the speech of women and children?
> Do people get annoyed because you misunderstand what they say?

"If you answered 'yes' to three or more of these questions," according to the National Institute, it's time you resolved to get a hearing evaluation.

Hearing Aids: "Eyeglasses" for the Ears? 10 JANUARY 1999

Some 10 percent of people in Western countries (plagued by noise and characterized by aging populations) are commonly said to suffer hearing loss.[2] That jibes with the estimate of 28 million Americans with hearing impairments, and some 2 million more in Australia and New Zealand, 3 million in Canada and in Scandinavia, 6 million each in Britain, France, and Italy, 9 million in Germany, and 15 million in Russia. Considering the rest of Europe, Asia, and the developing nations, with their younger populations and comparatively noise-free environments, we have a total of 300 million to 400 million humans with hearing loss. Yet only a little more than one-seventh of those 28 million Americans currently wear hearing aids. The rest either have not availed themselves of the technology or they keep their aids at home in the dresser drawer.

Why don't people with impaired hearing wear hearing aids as commonly as people with impaired vision wear glasses? Mark Ross offers several answers. In part, he believes, it is because of the stigma that attaches to hearing

2. The *New York Times,* as I mentioned earlier, has summarized a report by the National Institutes of Health that 28 million Americans are hard of hearing. The Better Hearing Institute reports three major studies estimating that between 25 and 28 million Americans—about 10 percent of us—suffer hearing loss. The institute indicates that the real number may be a tad higher, because such studies typically do not sample people in nursing and retirement homes. The National Center for Health Statistics report *Healthy People 2000* indicates that 8.5 percent of the population—23 million Americans in all—live with "significant hearing impairment." Most—18 million—are forty-five or over.

loss. We associate hearing aids (more than glasses) with aging and disability. Who wants to look and feel old and decrepit? Aided by cosmetics and plastic surgery, we spend fortunes denying our age. For many of us, to put on a visible hearing aid is to announce that we are aging. Everyone will know we're hard of hearing (gasp!—as if those who know us well would be shocked). Ironically, *not* wearing an aid may do even more to advertise that we are aging. In responding inappropriately or inattentively, people may seem rude, dim-witted, or closer to senility than any hearing aid could make them appear.

With the new generation of miniaturized, in-the-canal aids, the cosmetic barriers to wearing hearing aids are, however, coming down. The new aids are to hearing loss what contact lenses are to vision loss. Is President Clinton wearing his hearing aids? We don't know, because they are "completely in the canal."

A cost barrier does remain, especially for those interested in the new high-end digital aids. Yet middle-class people who balk at such a price tag may without blinking pay as much to buy a mid-sized rather than small new car, to fly to Honolulu for a two-week holiday, or to have cable television. As the market expands and the technology becomes mass-produced, we can hope that the price of processor chips for hearing aids will decline, as it has for desktop computers. Sixteen manufacturers have introduced digital aids or plan to do so soon (according to a recent *Hearing Journal* report), and the competition is sure to help. Moreover, Donna Sorkin, director of Self Help for Hard of Hearing People, foresees that health insurance providers and Medicare will offer reimbursement for hearing aids and audiological services as readily as they now reimburse those with vision loss for eyeglasses and those with impaired mobility for wheelchairs.

The psychologist in me senses additional reasons for our resistance. If the hearing loss experienced by all 28 million of us were abrupt—from one day to the next—we'd be stunned. Keenly aware of the sudden plunge, we would immediately seek a remedy, as do those who've lost hearing after a sudden explosion, illness, or accident. Instead, for most of us, hearing declines so gradually, so insidiously, that we perceive no difference from one month or year to the next. Oh, maybe we realize we're missing more than we did five or ten years ago. But we manage sufficiently well with most people most of the time that we attribute the occasional missed word to others' mumbling, slurring, or speaking too softly, or to background noise. They, of course, think the problem is with our hearing.

As I have noted before, we who are hard of hearing, aware of what we *do* hear, attribute our occasional hearing failures to the speaker or the noisy context. The person whom we haven't heard more likely thinks the problem is our poor hearing. These differing "attributions" reflect a pervasive tendency for human beings to explain their own behavior as a result of the situation, while attributing others' behavior to their traits. Social psychologists have observed the phenomenon in dozens of experiments. Imagine watching someone lecture. While your attention is focused on the lecturer, you may infer that this loquacious person is a natural extrovert. The lecturer, however, observes his or her own behavior in all kinds of situations—in the classroom, at home, in meetings—and so might say, "Me, outgoing? It all depends on the situation. In class or with friends, yes, I speak up. But at conventions or around strangers, I'm really rather shy." In the same way, I might say, "Me, hard of hearing? It all depends. With many people and in many situations I hear just fine."

Ergo, there's no need to accuse the hard of hearing of being in deep denial (perhaps related to fear of mortality).[3] Our resistance to acknowledging hearing loss can easily be explained by the imperceptible rate of erosion in our hearing, combined with our natural awareness of the way our responses vary according to the situation. Moreover, as I mentioned earlier, we sustain the illusion that we hear fine partly by not scoring as "misses" things we've never heard.

Once we put in a hearing aid, *then* we experience sudden change. Suddenly we find ourselves distracted by sounds that others have adapted to (and that we will again adapt to, with patience). But in the short run, the distractions are not pleasant. They're like the distracting visual world I experienced several months ago after receiving new monovision contact lenses—one for close-up reading (which blurred the world at a distance) and one for distance viewing (which blurred the type on pages). What an irritation—a half-blurred world wherever I looked.

Mysteriously, thanks to that wonderful human capac-

3. Authors of books on hearing loss seem to love the pop psychology idea of predictable stages in adjusting to loss, such as denial ("I'm getting along okay"), projection ("The acoustics in this room are lousy"), anger or depression ("If you're ashamed of me, why don't you go alone?"), and acceptance ("My hearing is failing, but I'm not"). Although people *do* take time to appreciate their need for hearing assistance, research psychologists report that people cope with loss in ways too varied to fit into any neat series of stages.

ity for adaptation, my world today seems clear as can be. If I close my left eye and look at a page, it's blurred. If I close my right eye and try to read a sign across the street, it's blurred. Yet when I look with both eyes, my brain somehow discounts the blurred image and gives me a clear world no matter where I look. Something like that happens with the ear, and that is why most dispensers of hearing aids allow a thirty-day trial period during which the cost is refundable, why New York State in 1998 legislated a forty-five-day test period, and why Self Help for Hard of Hearing People recommends a sixty-day trial period.

There is biological wisdom in our adapting to what is constant and attending to what is not. On entering your neighbor's living room, you smell an unpleasant odor. You wonder how she tolerates the stench, but within minutes you no longer notice it. When you jump into the swimming pool, you shiver and complain about how cold it is. A short while later a friend arrives, and you exclaim, "Come on in—the water's fine!" These examples illustrate sensory adaptation—our diminishing sensitivity to an unchanging stimulus. (To experience this phenomenon, move your watch up your wrist an inch: you will feel it—but only for a few moments.)

Adaptation enables us to focus our attention on *informative* changes in our environment without being distracted by the uninformative constant stimulation of garments, odors, and street noise. Our sensory receptors are alert to novelty; bore them with repetition, and they free our attention for more important things.

So, how can you adjust to harsh high-frequency sounds that you weren't hearing before, or to the odd, distracting sound of your voice? The answer is simple and sure. Just wear the hearing aid. If the initial stress is exhausting, gradually increase the number of hours you have it in. You can depend on adaptation. It is inevitable, so have patience.

How to Persuade? 15 JANUARY 1999

To family members and friends of the hard of hearing, I say, Please don't assume that we are inattentive or that we're ignoring you. If we interrupt conversation, don't consider us rude. We probably didn't realize that the other person hadn't finished speaking. If we resist hearing aids, don't assume that we're "in denial."

Still, it is natural to wonder how to motivate a parent, partner, or friend who *does* have a hearing problem to do something about it. Better Hearing Institute director Sergei Kochkin offers this advice:

> Start out with a soft sell approach by sharing information, for instance from the Better Hearing Institute, and stating, "You seem to be having difficulty with your hearing. Why don't you read this literature, it shows that nearly everyone with a hearing loss can be helped. I will be glad to go with you to have your hearing tested."
>
> Know that one of the most loving things you can do for a family member who denies [his or her] hearing loss is to confront [that person] using "tough love," much [as] you would with an alcoholic. For instance, "I suspect that you are embarrassed about your hearing loss. I am tired of repeating myself and I am uncomfortable being your hearing aid. From now on, I refuse to repeat myself over and over. Either you get your hearing tested and corrected or I will stop talking to you."

A less threatening version of this speech—one that "speaks the truth in love"—might combine reason and emotion:

> I love you, John. But I am tired of hearing the radio and television blare. I am weary of being misunderstood and ignored, and of repeating myself. I am tired of your interrupting when you don't realize that someone hasn't finished speaking. I am embarrassed for you. If only you realized—your hearing loss is more conspicuous than any hearing aid would be.
>
> So puhhl-le-e-ease would you—as a gift to both of us, the gift I most wish for from you—just get a hearing test. If our vision is blurry, we get our eyes checked and maybe get glasses. If our hearing is indistinct, we get our ears checked and maybe get 'glasses for the ears' . . . yes? Eyes or ears, it's no big deal, especially now that hearing aids come miniaturized and have the power to amplify speech more than they do background noise.

It may also help to use strategies for persuasion that have a basis in social psychology:

Use the foot-in-the-door technique. People who agree with a small request often later become more willing to comply with a bigger request. So you might ask, "Will you think about it?" Later: "Will you *seriously* consider doing it?" Still later: "I'd be glad to make an appointment for a free hearing test and go with you—or would you rather make it?"

To gain a concession, take advantage of the door in the face. Someone who has just turned down a large request (that is, who has slammed a door in your face) will often concede to a more modest second request. "Let's call right now." "No!" "Okay, how about after Christmas, when the kids have left?"

Stimulate active cognitive processing. Explore what hearing loss feels like. "How did you feel when you realized that you had interrupted Mary?" "Do you ever wish you could hear the doorbell or telephone from upstairs?"

Adapt the message to the person. Experiments have found that engaged, interested people respond best to logical arguments and evidence. "The new digital aids simulate natural hearing better than before by allowing for sound compression and frequency selection." Less interested people respond better to indirect cues, such as attractive comparisons. "President Clinton got hearing aids when he was younger than you are."

When all is said and done, family members and friends must also have patience. They can hope to shorten the average six-year span between the onset of adult hearing loss and the first visit to the audiologist. But it will take time for the loss to become sufficiently noticeable for us to get a hearing evaluation. And it takes time to adjust to the change not only in hearing but in identity.

7

Technology and Hearing Loss: Exciting Developments

Hearing Aids: Theme and Variations 20 JANUARY 1999

To prepare myself for the transition to the new generation of hearing aids, I've been surfing the Web and reading all I can about hearing aids. The basic theme is the same: all aids include a microphone, an amplifier, a speaker, and a battery. But they differ greatly, I've learned, in size, technology, and price.

SIZE VARIATIONS

Completely-in-the-canal (CIC) aids, such as Bill Clinton has chosen, are the smallest and least visible, yet they pack enough power for a wearer whose audiogram reveals a mild to moderately severe hearing loss.

In-the-canal (ITC) aids are also small, though they protrude slightly from the ear. They have enough power for wearers with a wide range of hearing loss. They fill the softer outer part of the ear canal, whereas the CIC aid extends so deep into the ear that the wearer must remove it by pulling on a filament extension cord. Both types capitalize on the natural amplification capabilities of the outer ear.

In-the-ear (ITE) aids come in a custom-made shell that fits securely into the outer ear with the speaker protruding into the canal. Their slightly larger size makes it possible to package some extra technology, such as dual-microphone systems and telecoils, which we'll discuss shortly.

The behind-the-ear (BTE) aid offers plenty of power and room for all the technology anyone might want.

A very few people with severe hearing loss use ultra-powerful body hearing aids, which are housed in a pocket case with an extension cord that connects to a speaker in the ear.

TECHNOLOGY VARIATIONS

Traditional (analog) aids offer a circuit that is not programmed or processed by a computer. Their purpose is to amplify sound, and the volume control lets the user decide how much sound comes through. Technologically the simplest, they are also the least expensive—often a thousand dollars or a little more a pair.

Programmable analog aids such as the one I currently have allow the audiologist to program the amplifier on a computer. Through digital technology, these aids instruct an analog amplifier about which sounds to amplify. Technologically and costwise, they occupy a middle ground between analog and fully digital aids and might cost $2,500 (give or take a few hundred) a pair.

Digital aids are to analog aids what compact disks are to records. Digitization converts incoming sounds to numbers, which a tiny microchip with the computing power of a desktop computer then analyzes and (unlike a C.D. player) reconstructs to suit the user's needs. Would it help to distinguish background noise from speech? to compress sound by making loud sounds softer and soft sounds louder? to shift duration or frequency of vowel or consonant sounds to address the individual type of hearing loss? to convert average, sloppy speech to clearer speech? As the software for effecting such changes improves, it can be incorporated into the hearing aid, much as we update our word-processing software every few years. When introduced, these sold for about $4,000 to $6,000 a pair. If the effectiveness of these new instruments attracts a great many new customers, the price should decline. As I write, digital aids are being marketed by Danavox (www. danavox.com), Oticon (www.oticonus.com), Resound (www.resound. com), Siemens (sat.eskatoo. de), Sonic Innovations (www.sonici.com), and Widex (www.widex.com). The competition among these companies to produce hearing assistance of ever higher quality at affordable prices shows the free market system at its best.

For those whose hearing loss is about the same at all frequencies, a traditional hearing aid may suffice. For those of us who want a hearing aid that can customize sound to meet our needs and filter out unwanted noise, the digital generation is here. More than four in five patients report satisfaction with these new aids, according to Sergei Kochkin—double the satisfaction level of twenty years ago, he suspects.

Some manufacturers claim that their microchip will perform millions of calculations per second, in multiple-frequency bands, to tailor the amplification to the individual hearing loss and level of auditory input. Some of these aids (though not the miniature CIC aids) also have two microphones: an omnidirectional microphone that detects background sound and a directional "zoom" microphone that, at the flick of a switch, picks up sound primarily from whatever direction the user is facing. By computing the difference between these inputs (and favoring sound that reaches the front microphone first), the hearing aid, like a coal miner's lamp, focuses where the head is pointed. This supposedly makes the new aids more speech-sensitive in noisy settings. (My new aids will have this feature. When I'm talking to Carol while a fan is running nearby, will the aids muffle the noise of the fan and amplify her voice, as is claimed?)

Enthusiasts of the new aids say that if your old hearing aids have been relegated to a drawer, you may want to revisit your audiologist. Yesterday's aids sounded like transistor radios; today's digital aids offer the clarity of a C.D. Yesterday's aids amplified all sound, including noise and sound in the frequencies we already heard well; today's aids can customize the output. Yesterday's aids were plagued by wind noise and feedback whistles; today's aids can be programmed not to produce such sound. Yesterday's aids had omnidirectional microphones; today's aids can have directional or multiple microphones. Yesterday's aids were bulky; today's are miniaturized. Yesterday's aids had volume controls to be contended with; today's aids are self-adjusting—they amplify soft sounds but not loud sounds, to suit our comfort level.

I can hardly wait to see whether all this technology really will, for me, make a noticeable difference.

Are Two Better than One? 25 JANUARY 1999

Another decision I face is whether to equip both my ears or to continue with only one aid, for the weaker ear. In my grandmother's day (my mother inherited her hearing loss from Grandmother before passing it on to me) this was an easy call. One unwieldy hearing aid with a separate battery, an amplifier, volume control, and a connecting cord was all any person wanted to wear and manage.

As hearing technology was modernized, audiologists came to see advantages to having two hearing aids but would often, as a compromise, fit a client with one in the hope that the benefits would supply the motivation to try a second. By buying just one aid in 1991, I cut the cost nearly in half—and reduced the hassle and the threat to my vanity. For me, one aid was better than none, but for some people the results are disappointing. For many, reports Mark Ross (via www.audiology.org), the benefits of two aids would have encouraged satisfaction and continued use.

Today, says Ross, "just about everybody . . . except many new and prospective hearing-aid users" agrees that two aids are better than one, for much the same reason that glasses with two lenses are superior to the monocles sometimes worn in old World War II movies. With two good ears:

We localize sound better.
We enjoy stereo hearing, and the aesthetic pleasure of acoustical depth.
We can rely on two working ears in acoustically stressful situations—"the better to hear you with, my dear."
We can make out sounds at lower volume (thanks to the doubled input).
We have a "good ear" on whichever side of our head someone speaks from.
We preclude any risk of "adult-onset auditory-sensory deprivation" (with the resulting ringing in the ears and

atrophied ability to process speech information from an unused ear—use it or lose it).

For these reasons, the consumer group Self Help for Hard of Hearing People agrees with audiologists that we have two ears for good reason and might as well make optimal use of them both. The rationale is persuasive.

Always Something New 4 FEBRUARY 1999

Hearing-aid technology is like the weather in Scotland: if you don't like it, wait an hour and it will change. The changes are gaining momentum, and they are exciting. In addition to digital hearing aids, many other "assistive-listening devices" are now available from hearing-assistance centers in major cities and from catalogues or on the Web (see the appendix or visit www.davidmyers.org). For those who no longer hear, there are also new signaling and displaying devices. Reading about this new technology staggers me. Mother was born twenty years too soon! On the Web and in other reading I discover:

Telephone assistance. I've already mentioned our family's failed experiment with TDDS, or TTYS,—devices that many deaf people find enormously helpful. And I've mentioned the volume-controllable phone amplifiers that easily connect between phone and handset, but that also now come built into many phones. Hearing-assistance centers will now also sell an in-line amplifier or amplified phone to permit increased clarity of speech by selectively amplifying high or low frequencies. Anyone with a family member who struggles to hear on a traditional phone need look no further for a Christmas or birthday gift idea.

For telephone assistance, telecoil (T-coil)-compatible phones complement the new hearing aids. When I switch them on, the telecoils in my digital hearing aids will receive electromagnetic information directly from any recently manufactured traditional or cordless phone. When the wearer is using the telecoils, the hearing aids' microphones are off. The net effect: room noise is reduced, and the digitally customized telephone sound will be broadcast to my ear.

These developments would have gladdened the heart of Alexander Graham Bell. Bell's mother was so hard of hearing that for many years she used a large black ear trumpet. As a young man, Bell taught in a school for teachers of the deaf. While working there, he met Mabel Hubbard, who had been deafened by scarlet fever at the age of five, and later he married her. One of his biographers, Jacqueline Langille, reports that "Bell always considered himself to be first and foremost a teacher of the deaf," and even after he had invented the telephone, "he continued to devote much of his time and energy to his projects for deaf children." Part of his legacy is the Alexander Graham Bell Association for the Deaf, which aims to empower those without hearing. It would therefore surely please him that, thanks to TDDs, phone amplifiers, and telecoils, his great invention now serves growing numbers of the deaf and hard of hearing.

F.M. and infrared systems. Even the best digital aids are not at their best when their microphones are far from a signal source—a person's voice, a television, an auditorium, or the speakers in a theater. If only there were binoculars for the ears that could reach out and pick up that sound at its source without the intervening sound degradation and noise—as if our ear were up close to the mouth or the television speaker. Well, now there are. My son Peter just gave me one such device for Christmas—a SONY F.M. system that has a) a transmitter that plugs into our television, and b) a wireless stereo headset that receives the signal. What a difference! With stereo sound piped directly into each ear, thanks to this miniature F.M. radio station, I can hear a depth of television sound that I never knew existed. (It's quite like sandwiching my head directly between two stereo speakers.) It's also easier to understand the accents on the British mysteries I love to watch. And because I can control my own volume (as with my older infrared system), Carol doesn't mind being in the room with me. The F.M. signal transmits clearly through walls, so I can also keep listening while I go make a cup of tea or fetch the newspaper.

The same technology is now in use in auditoriums, houses of worship, and theaters. Fortunately, many groups are now sensitive to the hard of hearing. They give their speakers microphones, ask them to repeat questions from the audience, and seat smaller groups at round or oval tables to enable each person to see all the others' faces. Large-area assistive-listening devices take the process a step further. They pick up the movie sound track or the speaker's voice at the source and transmit the signal (via F.M. radio, infrared light, or an induction-loop wire around the room) directly to special receivers or to a telecoil worn by the recipient. A person can wear an induction loop that receives an infrared signal and converts it to an electromagnetic signal to which the hearing-aid T-coil is sensitive. "I can't sufficiently emphasize how wonderful these systems are," reports Mark Ross from his own experience. Yesterday after church I approached a friend who was wearing a loop, and she said, "I'm classified as deaf, but this is the one place where, thanks to this loop, I can hear 99 percent of what's said!" Thanks to the Americans with Disabilities Act, all public accommodations must make the loops available and allow patrons to check out reception devices free of charge. Churches are not required to do so, but many, like my own, now offer the devices. Our college theater, for example, has enabled me to follow plays with much less strain, effort, and fatigue.

It is also possible to personalize an F.M. system. I can therefore imagine the day when I will do as some of the hard of hearing people already do: carry around a microphone or transmitter that can be pointed at a conversational partner or worn by their companion or by a lecturer whom they have approached before a class or meeting. In a noisy restaurant or on the street, Carol could clip my portable microphone to her blouse. My hearing aids would then receive the sound signal that comes out of her mouth, before it reverberates off hard surfaces and mingles with surrounding noise. In a department meeting, I could place one or two microphones in front of people on the other side of the table.

Hearing-assistance systems especially designed for air travel are also becoming available. Because F.M. radio and electromagnetic induction loops would interfere with the plane's own communication and electrical systems, the new hearing-aid travel systems use infrared light to convey the words of the pilot or flight attendant directly to the user's ear, but with automatic noise reduction. My other son, Andy, just gave me for Christmas another great toy, which I look forward to using on airplanes. It's noise-canceling earphones that I can plug into my cassette player or into a plane's sound system. The earphones block extraneous noise for two reasons—first, because their speakers are embedded in earplugs, and second, because each earphone contains a microphone that detects surrounding noise and generates a sound wave that cancels it. On a recent plane trip, music on the cassette player sounded as it would in my living room. The roar of the plane was blocked (unless I pushed a button to switch the incoming sound source).

Auto passengers can also look forward to hearing assistance. While in the backseat, perhaps of a minivan, have you ever had difficulty hearing the driver or front-seat passenger? If so, good news is on the horizon. Johnson Controls here in Holland, Michigan, a manufacturer of interior automotive systems, has developed a TravelCom communication system that will pick up voices from the front seat with an overhead mike, filter out ambient noise, and broadcast them through speakers. The resulting 66 percent voice magnification promises to make conversation more comfortable: no one has to shout, and the driver's eyes stay on the road.

All these assistive-listening devices increase the signal-to-noise ratio by doing what no hearing aid alone can do: putting a portable third ear—the microphone—close to the signal. The more I read about these assistive hearing systems, the more optimistic I feel about my own social future.

Captioning. If when you read "captioning" you thought of television, you were partly right. Larry Goldberg of the CPB/WGBH National Center for Accessible Media, who spoke recently at a hearing-technology research symposium, is hopeful about the future. Not only will high-definition (digital) television give us brighter, clearer pictures, but it will "greatly improve the look and reach of closed captions." ("Closed" captions appear only when a viewer opens them.) He anticipates, for example, that we will have the ability to select from as many as fifteen caption channels for each program—offering us verbatim or edited captions in any of several languages.

Although movie producers and theaters resist putting captions on movie screens, some are now introducing Rear Window captioning, visible only to those who want it. At the back of the theater a large screen displays captions in reversed letters. The patron then pulls up a sort of rearview mirror that catches the reflection for personal viewing. Because the mirror is clear plastic, it is possible to watch the movie right through it, or to make the reflections fall right below the screen. Disneyland and Disney World, the Epcot Center, and some IMAX and large-screen theaters around the country have already introduced Rear Window captioning.

Microsoft has also developed software that enables multimedia developers to offer closed captioning for video and audio clips, such as the ones it provides with its multimedia encyclopedia, *Encarta.* This technology should soon enable the developers who create the multimedia supplements for my textbooks to invite students who are deaf or hard of hearing to call up time-synchronized captions for the animations and media clips.

Looking to the future, the refinement of speech-recognition software holds great promise. It is now simple and effective enough to allow a seventy-two-year-old professor-friend in Scotland, who does not even have e-mail, to dictate and instantly print and fax me a memo, as he did yesterday. A few months back, Andy demonstrated DragonDictate's new continuous-speech-recognition software (it is no longer necessary for the speaker to put micropauses between words). I was amazed. Think of the possibilities. Already TDDs are being greatly speeded up because the dial-up intermediary may be repeating your words into speech-recognition software. And who needs an intermediary? If Mother were still alive, why shouldn't I be able (through either my software or the phone company's) to speak directly to her, with my words displayed both to me (for confirmation) and to her? This advance unquestionably lies in the near future—as do portable, in-home speech-translation systems that will fulfill my dream of more complete communication with people deafened late in life. I imagine that further in the future, we may have directional microphones that pick up ordinary conversation and display it—open-captioned—before our eyes.

That day may actually not lie so far in the future. After I had written this paragraph, someone told me about the Personal Captioner. Already being demonstrated in public presentations around the country, it consists of a pair of ordinary looking eyeglasses, embedded with a monitor that displays captions on the lenses. A person with hearing loss will be able to attend a first-run movie rather than waiting for a special captioned version and, thanks to wireless transmission and voice-recognition computer technology, see it captioned literally before his or her eyes. According to the developers, the words "seem to 'float' about eighteen inches in front of the eye. The captioning is always between the eye and the object being viewed. Turn or tilt the head, [and] the captioning remains within the line of sight" (www.multimediadesigns.com/pc.html).

Cochlear implants. By the time that fantasy is fulfilled, cochlear-implant technology may have obviated the need for it. The implant consists of a receiver and a sound processor placed in the bone behind the ear, with an electrode running to the cochlea, where it stimulates the hearing nerve. James Snow, director of the National Institute on Deafness and Other Communication Disorders, recently reported that a million Americans today could benefit from cochlear implants (which, as I wrote in the 2 February 1995 entry, are sometimes remarkably effective). Given the rate at which this hearing technology is developing, I have begun to believe one of my friends, who tells me, "You'll never go deaf, because by the time you would, implant technology will effectively solve the problem."

It could be. Michael Disher tells me that an 80-decibel hearing loss or a score of less than 45 percent on a sentence-comprehension test makes the patient a candidate for an implant.

> The best implant candidates are those recently deafened—ideally, [within] five years or less, but up to ten years of deafness is not a problem. The poorest candidates are adults deaf since birth or early childhood. In children the best candidates are the very young—two years or less if congenitally deaf. The earlier the implant, the better the result. The cost is about $40,000.

Studies have shown that deaf children who receive implants by the age of two develop age-appropriate language skills by six or seven. Late-deafened adults who are given implants soon after they have been deafened will function quite normally within six months to a year. New technology has contributed some very impressive improvements in performance.

Middle-ear implants. In Europe and the United States research and clinical trials are also being done on surgically implanted devices inside a healthy middle ear. Normal hearing aids amplify sound before it reaches the middle ear. The implants amplify the movement of the tiny bones within the middle ear. One device detects the sound vibrations transmitted by the bone attached to the back of the eardrum and converts the vibrations into electrical signals. These signals are then amplified, filtered, and reapplied as mechanical vibrations to the stapes bone that connects with the inner ear. (For examples, see www.symphonix.com and www.stcroixmedical.com.)

Alerting devices. In the meantime, for people who cannot afford implants or people for whom the implants don't work, hearing-assistance centers also offer alerting devices. For people who don't hear alarms, there are bedshakers, vibrating wrist alarms, and flashing lights. Flashing lights can also alert the deaf to the ringing of a doorbell, smoke alarm, telephone, or pager. These devices can also transmit an alert (often a vibration) wherever in the house a person happens to be. In a hotel room, a light connected to the door knocker can be affixed to the inside of the door. General Motors will help deaf car buyers pay for an emergency alert response system (EARS) that alerts them when an emergency vehicle is approaching. For those who sometimes leave a turn signal on, a flashing light on the dashboard can be triggered after fifteen seconds without braking (for the turn) have passed.

The Internet. One other marvelous communication technology is ours now, and that is our new capacity to glean information and communicate with one another via the Internet. How my life has changed! I now receive only occasional personal letters, fewer faxes than only recently was the case, many fewer disruptive phone calls at work—and more than 5,000 personal e-mail messages a year (often several an hour during prime working hours). E-mail is a bane, but even more it's a blessing . . . not only because communication takes place at my convenience but also because I can understand it completely, without any strain.

Only recently did I learn from articles in *Hearing Health* and the *New York Times* that Vinton Cerf, co-developer of the Internet, has a severe hearing loss. Partly because of this, Cerf was comfortable with text messages, which he made part of the early Internet system. Surrounded by the whirring fans of computers, Cerf had a hard time hearing technical information over the phone and found e-mail communication "a relief." In the early 1990s, her husband's Internet helped Sigrid Cerf research cochlear implants for her own use. Using a TDD service, she could not receive a return call from the Johns Hopkins University physician to whom her research had directed her. So she e-mailed the doctor, got a response the next day, and today hears with the help of an implant.

Thanks to Vinton Cerf and others, the deaf and hard

of hearing are benefiting even more than the hearing from the Internet. E-mail, Web surfing, and on-line chats level the playing field. For the hearing and nonhearing, "it's a great equalizer," reflects Cerf. How fortunate I am that I was not born thirty years earlier!

The Time Has Come 16 FEBRUARY 1999

The new technology is now available, and today my audiologist had me in to make ear molds—the first step in being fitted with aids. My audiologist also took the opportunity to offer helpful feedback on the manuscript for this book. "Don't overpromise what the new technology can accomplish," he cautioned. "Remember how, earlier, you outlined the ear's fantastic feats. No prosthesis will ever duplicate that normal function. If you raise expectations too high, people may be disappointed with even the best aids." I get the sense that he's also cautiously trying to moderate my expectations.

But then again, positive expectations may boost satisfaction. That is what University of Iowa professor Ruth Bentler reports in a recent issue of the *Hearing Journal.* She and her merry prankster associates had people alternately try two digital aids for a month each, but labeled one "digital . . . with CD quality sound, microprocessor sound filtering, etc.," and the other analog. At the end of the trial, most subjects preferred whichever aid was hyped as digital. Even when subjects were given the same aid twice, they preferred a "digital" over an "analog" aid (although, not surprisingly, their speech-perception scores with the two aids did not vary).

Bentler does, however, report that in most clinical trials comparing hearing enhanced by digital aids with unaided hearing and with hearing with conventional aids, the "predominant finding has been improved hearing."

Where the Fingers Do the Talking 18 FEBRUARY 1999

This afternoon, while in Washington, D.C., I had my first immersion into the deaf world when I was invited to lunch with the Gallaudet University psychology department and then to visit a classroom. Gallaudet's undergraduate students are all deaf, at least to the point of having significant difficulty in a hearing world. Although two-thirds of the faculty are hearing, all new faculty who are nonsigners are immediately put into a Sign immersion program and must achieve fluency in signing before receiving tenure. (Sign translators are available during their transition.)

This experience of a new culture reminded me of my wide-eyed curiosity during the first days of our year in Scotland. Some observations and answers to my questions:

- Everyone I spoke with during my visit, whether hearing or not, signed while speaking, even if only to me. Was this simply automatic behavior in that setting? Or was it, as I assumed, sensitivity to any others around the table who might wish to eavesdrop or join in the conversation? It was both, my host later explained: "There's a *really* strong message from the time you arrive here that you should *always* sign when you speak, so that deaf people have equal access. Talking without signing is like whispering in front of someone else."

- How does the human brain accomplish simultaneous speaking and signing? Given the impossibility, discussed earlier, of devoting attention to two sources simultaneously, does signing occur unconsciously, while the person is paying conscious attention to the spoken words? How do you speak two languages at the same time? That's not really how it works, my hosts explained. You would be speaking English and signing in English at the same time. (The signs for English and ASL words are essentially the same; it is their grammar that differs.) When you are signing ASL, you are using the grammar of ASL. To my ear, ASL, when literally translated into spoken English, sounds like English ordered according to the grammar of another language. "Finish me not yet" (English translation: I'm not finished yet"). "Buy house white, country, beautiful" (I bought a white house in the country. It's beautiful"). The examples were offered by a faculty member who, as the hearing child of deaf parents, has native fluency in both languages. Another said it reminded him of when he tried to translate German into English, word for word, "and ended up with gibberish."
- "Deaf of deaf" students are in the minority among deaf people and among Gallaudet students. (Most deaf students, whether deaf from birth or deafened later, have hearing parents.) Nevertheless, these deaf of deaf students are the social elite year after year—the Gallaudet student leaders. Why? "This is a university for deaf people, and they're the deafest we have."
- "Are the advances in cochlear-implant technology for children seen here as a threat to the deaf culture?" I asked. Indeed, came the answer, and the number of cochlear implants among middle-class deaf children is "exploding." Parents, doctors, and audiologists who advocate implants are promoting children's integration into the hearing world and thus are generally not sup-

portive of signing. "Have you known of any *deaf* parents who have sought to obtain an implant for their deaf child?" My companions looked at each other and agreed: they were unaware of such a case.

- My faculty host, whose long-standing invitation to come to Gallaudet had prompted my visit, invited me to return when I had time to give my talk on happiness. "Do you give your visiting speakers any special instructions?" I wondered. "Yes. We tell them to speak as they normally would, to look at their audience, not their interpreter, and to pause to let people read slides." Well, of course, it dawned on me: a hearing audience can listen and look simultaneously. A deaf audience must digest the spoken explanation and the slides sequentially.
- I sensed that I was the only person struggling to catch the signed-and-spoken lunch table conversation. Neither the deaf nor the fully hearing had any difficulty. As the only one in that in-between land—ignorant of Sign yet unable to hear many of the spoken words—I strained to hear, sometimes asking people to repeat and sometimes letting the missed remark go by.
- When I observed that it was impossible to use a knife and fork and sign at the same time, I asked whether eating interfered with communication. "Ah, but we can sign with our mouths full!"

Visiting an art history class was also a revealing experience. The first thing that struck me when I walked in was the wonderful classroom architecture. At Hope College, I have long argued, the typical classroom seating is out of synch with the pedagogical principles we espouse. We promise instructor-led classes with lots of animated discussion. But our classrooms—most of which have straight rows of chairs facing a talking head—give students minimal visual access to one another. Not so at Gallaudet, where new classrooms, for obvious reasons, are designed to make it easy for students to see one another. In the class I visited, one U-shaped table was surrounded by a second elevated U-shaped table—precisely the sort of classroom design that should predominate at any liberal arts college.

And what an animated, if silent, discussion took place about the differences between French and German Expressionism. As the instructor threw out questions, several students would often begin answering at once. (One person's signing doesn't instantly cancel out another's, the way one speaking voice inhibits another.) Observing all this impressed on me anew how rich, intricate, efficient, and effortless signed communication can be. But if you consider how effortlessly words roll out of the mouth, how syllables form with precise tongue rolls and lip movements, how words instantly order themselves in syntax, why should the fluid finger, hand, and arm gestures of the signer be any less smooth? Moreover, reports Michael Corballis in *American Scientist* (March–April 1999), human language may have evolved from hand signals. If so, it's no wonder that gestures survive as part of hearing people's speech, even when they are talking on the phone. And it's no wonder that signing developed among deaf people as an alternative to speech.

As students made presentations to the class, I occasionally noticed the sort of trivial grammatical error on their slides that might be made by anyone who had learned English as a second language ("He born on June 12." "He had large number of hundred self-portraits"). But my overwhelming impression was of how effective this bilingual, hearing instructor was (for my sake, she spoke that day as well as signed, and the interpreter remained at my side) and especially how animated, interested, and intelligent the students were. I think most art history instructors would have been envious.

One other small observation: at Gallaudet, "whispers" and offhand comments, unless made furtively or under the table, do not remain private. My host recalled once noticing two students "planning a party, right down to who would pick up the keg. I asked, in front of the class, whether they were planning to invite the whole class to their party. Oh, were they embarrassed! They didn't talk in my class again."

Liking Deaf Better? 26 FEBRUARY 1999

Four hours ago my ears were stuffed with $4,400 of today's technology. After inserting the aids and temporarily attaching them to his desktop computer, my audiologist ran a test, electronically read my stored audiogram, and then programmed the aids accordingly. Soft, low sounds are enhanced by as much as 28 decibels in the left ear, loud or high sounds much less. These in-the-ear aids are somewhat smaller than the hearing aids I have had, but they protrude more than I had anticipated—and even more than Ed, my audiologist, would like ("because you have a shallow ear bowl").

"Well," I tell Ed, "a guy of fifty-six cares more about function than about cosmetics. As a teen, appearance mattered so much. Now I often look in the mirror during a late-morning bathroom stop and realize that I've neglected to comb my hair." "Yeah, well, you're a college professor," Ed replies, implying that most people do worry about their appearance. In fact, I do wish the aids weren't quite so obvious.

My immediate reaction when Ed switches on the new aids is much the same as my reaction to the previous technology eight years ago. My voice—it's so loud! (Carol tells me I often speak too loudly. Perhaps that problem will quickly be solved.) When I get into my car, the door slams, the seat belt locks noisily, and the blinker signal seems obnoxiously loud. And the radio—someone left it blaring! All this reminds me of the remark by a child of a family friend, shortly after he had received a cochlear implant: "Daddy, I think I like deaf better."

Then I recalled this week's frustrating faculty meeting, where I had missed most of a lively debate. (A supportive colleague later summarized it for me.) Maybe, on second thought, I don't like hard of hearing better.

Zoom, Zoom 27 FEBRUARY 1999

This weekend I'm attending a "communitarian summit" in Washington, D.C. At one session the speaker's voices seemed so strong that I assumed the room must be equipped with microphones, but later I learned that it was not. The amplification devices were in my ears. Although the applause was irritatingly loud, I loved being able to hear *all* the questions and comments from the audience. The only stressful moment came when I stood up to ask a question and felt overwhelmed by my own voice (it came out fine, but the shock of it brought beads of perspiration to my face).

The aids come with a tiny, protruding push button that allows me to switch the sound from "basic" to "directional" to "telecoil" (with one, two, or three beeps—heard only by me—to confirm the setting). On "basic" I can hear people equally well whether they are in front of me or beside or behind me. On "telecoil" the aids become earplugs—blocking all sound except for that transmitted by a phone receiver or a neck loop. A little test at a pay phone in a noisy room suggested that I could probably hear better than fully hearing people—because I hear only what comes from the phone.

On "directional" I am supposed to hear someone in front of me noticeably better, while the sound from other directions is reduced. And I do! At a noisy cocktail party I switched on "directional," and the speech of the person I was looking at came across as clear as a bell. While waiting to have a word with a syndicated columnist, I found myself able—if I faced him—to make out his words from a certain distance as he finished talking to someone else, almost as if I were eavesdropping. At dinner, with 250 people talking and a loud band playing, I again turned on the directional mike and had absolutely no problem understanding my companions on either side (one of whom moved to sit closer to me because *she* was having trouble hearing). Although the background noise is still quite audible, my conversational partner's voice comes through clearly amid the surrounding hubbub. This is remarkable! And a new study in the *Journal of American Academy of Audiology* (March 1999) confirms the advantage to the listener of directional microphones, especially in noisy situations—precisely where people with hearing loss need the most help.

When I told Carol about the directional capability of

the new hearing aids she joked that she and the kids would have to watch what they say to each other about me, now that they'll no longer be out of my earshot. That reminds me of the joke about the elderly man whose audiologist inquires whether the family is pleased by the old fellow's much improved hearing, now that he has the new aids. "Oh, I haven't told my family yet. I just sit around and listen to their conversation. I've already changed my will three times!"

If anything, the dramatic improvement in the signal-to-noise ratio exceeds my expectations. Reluctant hearing-aid wearers could hardly have a better incentive to take their aids out of the drawer each morning than a breakthrough of this magnitude. Our local paper quotes a man who is severely hard of hearing and has just purchased the same technology: "This is absolutely without reservation the best hearing device I've ever worn! This technology allows me to hear things I couldn't hear before. It's wonderful."

Think how far we have come from a century ago, when our great-great-grandparents who were hard of hearing had nothing more than an ear horn or speaking tube to funnel sound to their ears; and from a half century ago, when my grandmother carried a clumsy hearing device the size of a pack of cigarettes and had to change a battery every two or three days to keep the vacuum tubes functioning.

Adapting — 3 MARCH 1999

In more and more situations where hearing used to be a challenge, I now love listening, thanks to this new technology . . . but how much less I enjoy talking! For an extrovert who sometimes (Carol says) blurts things out inappropriately, talking less may not be a bad thing. She tells me that my voice is definitely softer.

That modulation may last, but I suspect that my reluctance to speak will not. I find that when I start talking, I'm often conscious of my voice, but as the conversation picks up momentum, I become engrossed and stop feeling self-conscious. Given our ability to adapt to changing visual and auditory situations, I suspect that even the initial self-consciousness will gradually subside.

A Noisy Noise Annoys an Oyster and Afflicts a Cochlea

2 MAY 1999

The *intensity* and the *duration* of noise together determine the damage noise will do. The louder the noise, the less time it is safe to listen to it. Brief exposure to extremely intense sounds, such as nearby gunfire, can damage the hair cells of the inner ear. As a child, Marilyn Mobley, whose father was a gunsmith, spent her summers practice-shooting at bales of hay. Her hearing, as a consequence, was severely affected, according to *U.S. News and World Report.* Prolonged exposure to intense sounds, such as amplified music, can also damage hair cells. Nancy Nadler, director of the Noise Center at New York's Center for the League for the Hard of Hearing, likens hair cells to the fibers of a shag carpet. After being walked on, the fibers will revive with a vacuuming. But if a heavy piece of furniture is placed on the carpet for a prolonged period, the fibers may never rebound.

Small wonder that with industrialization, power tools, and noisy recreational activities such as snowmobiling, the proportion of forty-five- to sixty-four-year-old Americans who "cannot hear and understand normal speech" shot up by 87 percent in the two decades following 1971 (according to National Health Interview Surveys). Paradoxically, even health clubs and fitness spas—which commonly blare 100-decibel music—may be damaging their patrons' auditory health. They might take a cue from Pete Townshend of the Who, who sent Hearing Education and Awareness for Rockers a check for $10,000, acknowledging his own hearing loss.

As a general rule, says Ross Roeser, former president of the Better Hearing Institute (www.betterhearing.org), if you can't talk over a noise, then you should consider it potentially harmful, especially if it is prolonged. People who spend their days behind a power mower or a jack hammer should be wearing earplugs. For those who can do so, walking away from ear-splitting racket is a safer expedient than inserting earplugs. A ringing in the ears after exposure to loud machinery or music is a sign of possible damage to the hair cells. As pain alerts us to possible bodily harm, ringing in the ears alerts us to a potential hearing problem. "Condoms or, safer yet, abstinence," say youth sex educators. "Earplugs or, safer yet, walk away," say hearing educators.

John Wheeler, president of the Deafness Research Foundation (www.drf.org), explains, "We want to shift public attitudes . . . to the belief that each person's hearing should be protected from noise trauma throughout

Figure 7.1 The Year 2010

To stimulate our thinking, imagine America's hearing health scene in 2010. Changes like these are possible, and many will occur:

Ninety-eight percent of newborns receive screening. Four thousand babies per year get implants, along with 2,000 more children and teens. The average age of implantation is nine months and is trending younger. Another 8,000 newborns are receiving hearing aids. Over 30,000 adults are receiving implants, a figure that is also increasing annually.

The annual US market for hearing aids has quadrupled since 1999 because hearing aids so enhance hearing, especially for listening to music, that they are fashionable. Hearing aid "stigma" is forgotten.

A simple home-based, self-administered audiology exam is used by over 30 million families each year. The exam uses the Internet and audio connection to the computer, tripling 1999's demand for audiological services, since people want to confirm the home-test and seek hearing devices. Because the test uncovers cases where otitis media has gone undiagnosed and is damaging hearing, the demand for otological services has nearly doubled since 1999.

The need for speech therapists has doubled since 1999, spurred by growth in home-tests and demand for implants. A home-test for otitis media is available by prescription. Almost all tinnitus can be suppressed by medical intervention in the brain's processing centers, and controls on toxic noise are slowing the incidence of hearing loss, tinnitus and hyperacusis.

The Environmental Protection Agency in Washington, D.C., is issuing its proposed Toxic Noise Regulations after a period of notice and comment. They cover point and area sources of toxic noise, stationary and mobile sources, and all areas outside the workplace.

Gallaudet University receives Congressional approval to expand enrollment of non-US students to 80 percent, in stages, between 2010 and 2020, so that Gallaudet can serve students from countries where hearing aids and cochlear implants are not available to the bulk of the population. This shift compensates for the declining enrollment of US students due to newborn screening and intervention via hearing aids or implants. The legislation expands the Washington campus and deploys faculty and graduates to create campuses in Africa, Latin America, China, India, and Eastern Europe; and funds Gallaudet through the World Bank and the US Agency for International Development.

Source: Reprinted by permission from John Wheeler, "The Year 2010," *Hearing Health*, January–February 2000, p. 11. John Wheeler is president and CEO of the Deafness Research Foundation, which sponsors Hear US, the National Campaign for Hearing Health.

life. . . . We want children to grow up taking as much care of their hearing as they now take for their teeth, creating a lifetime habit of avoiding, blocking or eliminating unnecessary sonic damage. There is tooth decay; there is also 'hearing decay.' We use seatbelts and keep safe vehicle speeds; we can use ear plugs and keep safe sound levels." If we can support new bioelectronic breakthroughs by greatly increasing the currently meager public funding for research into hearing loss, "*the end of all hearing loss is in reach,*" Wheeler declares. More realistically and immediately, he proposes a national goal of halving the rate of hearing loss by around the year 2000 (see also Figure 7.1).

The Deaf Sentry 17 MAY 1999

Yesterday evening, after a thunderstorm knocked out the power in our neighborhood, Carol and I headed to bed early. Just as we were drifting off to sleep, she roused herself. "What was that?"

Hearing nothing, I tried to elicit from her whether the noise had come from outside or inside. Without answering, Carol uttered something between a gasp of panic and a muffled scream—we had an intruder in the house! Both of us sat bolt upright, though I still had no idea what kind of threat we were facing. Finally I heard something, too—a familiar voice calling up the stairs. It was our son Andy. Assuming we'd still be up, he had come over from his nearby apartment to collect a flashlight.

"I guess we won't depend on you to detect intruders," Carol reflected afterward. Oh, well, she can be our ears.

Frustration and Aggression 20 MAY 1999

Although I'm keenly aware of the frustrations caused by hearing impairment, I was stunned by McCay Vernon and Sheldon Greenberg's conclusions in an article reviewing new research, "Violence in Deaf and Hard-of-Hearing People," in the fall 1999 issue of *Aggression and Violent Behavior:* "A clear and significant positive correlation exists" between hearing loss and violence. Vernon and Greenberg recount recent cases in which deaf people have committed murder, including that of John Kemink, the doctor with whom I had corresponded (as I wrote in my entry of 9 November 1992). Of course, with some 20 thousand homicides annually in the United States, it is inevitable that deaf people will be among the perpetrators. More intriguing is the authors' report that people with hearing impairments are overrepresented in prisons. In screenings of prison inmates in Michigan, Ohio, Maryland, and Wisconsin, it was found that roughly three in ten had significant hearing loss.

Vernon and Greenberg conjecture that the physical, social, and economic challenges of being deaf or hard of hearing create "frustration which tends to manifest [itself] in disproportionate aggression, violence, and hostility." It will take a lot more research to sort out the genetic, educational, economic, and psychological roots of this violence. In general, however, the link between frustration and aggression is well established. The 99 percent of the deaf and hard of hearing who are not overtly violent may therefore want to remain alert to other aggressive tendencies in themselves. If physical aggression isn't their style, they may respond to frustration with heightened verbal aggressiveness or plain old crabbiness.

Open to Closed Captions 28 JUNE 1999

As Andy and I sat down to watch *Chariots of Fire* on his new DVD player, he asked whether I'd like the captioning turned on. Sure, I said, knowing that without it I'd be struggling to decipher the different British accents. The captioning proved so helpful that this weekend, when catching up on my favorite British television mysteries on PBS and A&E, I again opened the closed captioning (which to my surprise worked on videotaped as well as broadcast programs).

Closed captioning is wonderful. With the help of the captions, I caught all the dialogue, even muttered Cockney phrases. Lyrics to songs are now intelligible, and the captioning also describes nonverbal nuances I would otherwise miss (a buzzing fly, a groan). Primed by the captions, I could even understand the *spoken* dialogue without turning the sound up too much. (Speech suddenly becomes clearer when you know what words to expect.)

The captions were so helpful—and would be for many fully hearing people when they are listening to accented speech, as well—that I feel one regret: If only it hadn't taken me so long to discover how useful the captions are! Having associated captioning with Mother, who was deaf, I hadn't realized that captions can be a resource for the hearing, too.

Rock and Ring 3 AUGUST 1999

A report just released by Britain's Royal National Institute for Deaf People blames loud music, now louder than ever, for an alarming rise in hearing loss. Digital technology allows people to play music at concerts and on C.D.'s at much higher volumes without distortion. The result, according to a synopsis in today's London *Times,* is that "three times as many young people are exposed to dangerous sound levels today as in the early 1980s." One British study found that 73 percent of rock concert fans experience dulled hearing, tinnitus, or both immediately afterward. "Tests have shown that 44 percent of those who attend rock concerts once a month have hearing difficulties."

Why not do today's kids a huge favor and make information about hearing an essential part of their health education curriculum? Listening to loud music can have devastating repercussions.

From the Speaker's Mouth to My Head 5 AUGUST 1999

My instantaneous reaction yesterday evening to my first experience with telecoil technology in a public setting was one of amazement. About 300 people were attending a dignified evening vespers service within the high stone walls of the 800-year-old restored abbey on Scotland's remote Isle of Iona. The tiny Atlantic island is known to millions as the place where in A.D. 563 St. Columba came over from Ireland to establish a Celtic Christian community and begin his work of establishing churches in this country (which means that he is to Scotland roughly what St. Patrick is to Ireland).

The sound of singing, as it reverberates off the hard stone walls of the abbey, takes on richness and depth. As I knew from previous visits here, though, hearing spoken words, even over the P.A. system, can be a challenge. Or it was, until Carol noticed an obscure sign advising hearing-aid wearers to switch on their T-coils. When I did so, the transformation in the sound was immediate and dramatic. Suddenly the babble of people awaiting the start of the service was replaced by the pure harmonies of the musicians—whom I had not even heard—playing in front of microphones across the abbey. My mouth literally fell open. It was like listening to a C.D. over a headset.

When the liturgy began, my astonishment remained unabated. The leader's words seemed to travel directly from her microphone to the center of my head (with the volume varying somewhat depending on which direction I was facing). Her voice could not have been more distinct. If I pulled the hearing aids out, I could barely understand her. At either of the other hearing-aid settings, the sound improved, but was somewhat echoing.

Afterward, our daughter Laura (who is volunteering with the Iona Community that occupies the abbey and a campsite on the adjacent island of Mull) introduced me to the abbey warden and to the current leader of the community. They received my thanks with obvious pleasure, and one of them remarked that I probably heard the spoken word more clearly than most. How true!

This is too good not to become routinely available in public places. The more the technology is in use (and therefore becomes appreciated), the more it will become available—even, I foresee, in airports and on trains and buses. Imagine: for many this would bring an enormous reduction in confusion (Was the gate agent saying something about why we aren't boarding?), anxiety, and misunderstanding (the train for Edinburgh is leaving from Track 6 . . . I'm pretty sure they said).

Divulging Difficulties Diminishes Distress

20 AUGUST 1999

At dinner last night, discussion of my hearing loss prompted a good Scottish friend to remind me that he had completely lost the hearing in one ear after having surgery, necessitated by Ménière's disease. "With hearing in only one ear, don't you have trouble locating sounds?" I wondered.

"Yes! Someone calls my name and I have no idea where the person is. 'Where are you?' I ask. 'Here,' comes the reply. '*Where?*' I plead, embarrassed and straining to locate the person. 'Here!' comes the reply again. It's horrible."

But an even more stressful experience soon after he had lost his hearing persuaded him to divulge his hearing loss openly from then on. As a guest minister at Crathie Church across the road from Balmoral Castle, he was invited to spend the weekend with the royal family during their annual sojourn in Scotland. At dinner the first evening he was seated between Queen Elizabeth and her lady-in-waiting, so that his good ear was toward the queen. After some minutes in conversation with her, he turned and found that the lady-in-waiting had been speaking to him without his having heard anything. So he turned to face her. He soon realized with dismay that he now had his back to the queen and was unable to hear and respond appropriately to her. Turning repeatedly to monitor the conversation on both sides proved exhausting. "If only I had not tried to hide my problem, and had instead just said to the woman on my right, 'You should know that I am deaf in this ear, so if you want my attention, just touch my arm.'"

Ever since then, he has made it a practice to do as all of us with hearing loss should do: alleviate his tension and his conversational partners' frustration by disclosing his difficulty. As he explained to his ministerial colleagues when he chaired a meeting shortly thereafter, "You should know that I have one deaf ear, and I intend to use it!"

An Identity for the Hard of Hearing 24 SEPTEMBER 1999

If my day at Gallaudet was my first immersion in deaf culture, today was my first immersion in the culture of the hard of hearing (HOH). I gathered with one hundred other Michiganders at a state SHHH conference. The experience of being in a room full of people like me was perhaps something like that of an adopted American child of Korean parentage when first surrounded by other Koreans. No self-consciousness about hearing aids or hearing difficulties here!

I came full of curiosity. I wondered, for example, how HOH people would communicate at such a meeting. The answer is, first of all, by being sensitive to people's needs. "Can everyone hear me?" began one speaker, with a twist of unintentional irony. "Is anyone having trouble hearing me?"

For the two deaf people, there were ASL interpreters. For most of the rest of us—those with hearing aids—microphones had been provided, of course, but also infrared assistive devices (available with either headsets or T-coil loops), and we were surrounded by an electromagnetic audioloop. The infrared devices, now available with hiss-free digital transmission, featured clear sound and volume control but needed to be pointed at the transmitter. The loop system in the room worked without a hitch, uninterrupted by passersby or listeners' shifts in position. The sound it produced was so clear, in fact, that I savored it with a mild feeling of ecstasy.

For the profoundly hard of hearing, every spoken word appeared on a giant screen displaying computer-assisted real-time transcription (CART), also called stenocaptioning or real-time captioning. The stenographer, who used to accompany a mainstreamed deaf child to school each day, now captions news broadcasts for a Detroit television station from her home. ("No one does it from the station," she told me.) Her transcriptions precisely reflected the spoken words, lagging behind them by a mere three words or so. Speakers average 150 words a minute and, to graduate after two or more years of training, a stenographer-captioner must transcribe better than 230 words per minute. In speed contests, some approach 300 words a minute.

Speaking on the identity of the hard of hearing, SHHH acting executive director Brenda Battat noted that the media and the general public equate hearing assistance during public events with ASL interpretation. In so doing, they lump millions of HOH and late-deafened people in with the 300 to 400 thousand or so who use ASL. So we commonly have interpreters for major public events but not loop systems or CART for the many additional people who might benefit from assistance. One-third of all hearing-aid wearers now have T-coils, we were told, and the proportion is surely rising. Moreover, one hearing-assistance vendor told me, he would install a loop system in any church sanctuary or theater for no more than $250. "After all, it takes half a day, no matter how big the room is."

The reason such systems are not installed more often, explained Brenda Battat, is that unlike the deaf, who have an identity and the pride that accompanies it, we don't. We have shame. And we are also more dispersed—indeed, we want to be part of the mainstream. Because of our shame and our dispersal and our diversity, we are invisible. We are silent and passive rather than vocal. We suffer the stress and isolation of impoverished communication and diminished relationships. We are not comfortable in deaf culture—we are more hearing than deaf—yet we are not completely comfortable in hearing culture. And so we make do with minimal advocacy for our needs.

By offering an identity to the HOH and serving as an advocate for them, SHHH aims to change that. Thanks to the tireless advocacy of people like Brenda Battat, herself too hard of hearing to use a normal phone comfortably, assistive systems are now mandated for new public structures in the United States. School systems now provide effective communication to children with hearing loss. All new televisions have chips that decode captions. All new phones are T-coil–compatible. Within the next decade, all new television programs and 75 percent of reruns will be captioned. And beginning in 2000, all phones will be manufactured with a volume control.

From Silence to Sound 24 SEPTEMBER 1999

A surprising number of the adults at this conference—about ten—were wired for sound with cochlear implants.

I talked with fifty-year-old Brian Sheridan, who two and a half years ago was at his wits end. Brian explained that by the age of ten he had normal hearing at low frequencies, significant loss at 2,000 hertz, and no hearing in ranges above that. His hearing loss presented day-to-day difficulties but did not preclude his attending law school with no hearing aids and becoming an attorney. During the 1990s, however, further decline motivated him to get progressively more powerful and sophisticated hearing aids.

Seeing the direction in which things where headed, Brian, along with his wife and his secretary, in 1993 took classes in Exact Signed English (ESE). Finding it "very hard to learn, I set up a system in my office where my secretary could listen in on calls and type a sort of shorthand transcript in real time on my computer to allow me to respond." He researched "accommodations for the hearing-impaired in state courts" and wrote up his findings for the state bar journal; he was also the first to argue to a case in his federal circuit court with the assistance of real-time captioning. By 1996, "most of the dialogue around me was taking place in a language I no longer understood: spoken English. I felt like Moses in Exodus 2:22: 'I have been a stranger in a strange land.'"

By 1996, the FDA had declared that people who were severely hard of hearing (roughly, those unable to use an amplified telephone) were eligible for implants. When Sheridan got in contact with the University of Michigan's Cochlear Implant Center in 1996, he learned that to qualify he must first undergo screening. He would take a test in which sentences were to be read to him by an unseen speaker. "If I scored over 40 percent, then I would not be an implant candidate. The night before the test I became nervous that I would fail (in other words, pass), so I asked my wife to read me sentences at random from *National Geographic* while I sat with my back to her. After a period of silence, I turned around and asked, 'Have you started yet?' only to find out that she had already read several sentences. Thus prepared, I went into the test with great confidence and got less than the cutoff."

On 5 January 1997, then, Brian underwent surgery at the University of Michigan Medical Center, a leading center for implant surgery (www.med.umich.edu/oto/ci). Blue Cross paid for the $40,000 of surgery and equipment—"everything up to when they switched it on" (the cost of all the audiological support services he needed after that had to be paid for out of pocket).

When the implant was activated on 5 February, "the biggest surprise was that speech was comprehensible. Since I had never heard most speech frequencies, my initial impression, however, was that everyone's voice sounded incredibly high-pitched." Brian's journey from silence to sound also introduced him to "fascinating new aspects of the world. The sound on the roof of our van as we left the implant center after the first day was a sound I had never heard, and I had to ask what it was. The sound of windshield wipers was completely new to me, as well as the warning beeps when the car lights are left on. When my secretary came into the office the first day after my activation, she said good morning to me from outside my office and was absolutely flabbergasted when I responded, 'Good morning!' to her."

Brian was told that adapting to an implant is a five-year process. He still has trouble recognizing voices. "I sometimes can't tell whether a voice is male or female. When I call home, I'm often unsure if my wife or one of my daughters has answered. Once I know who it is, the sound 'clicks' for me and it sounds like a man or woman. If I don't know who it is, the sound seems neutral, although the content is usually clear." But as time goes on, he is getting better at guessing the gender of unseen speakers.

Nowadays, he talks easily on the phone. As I bombarded him with questions, he didn't ask to have one word repeated. "Sounds as if this has made a huge difference in your life," I observed. Brian replied: "You should talk to my family and my office staff. My hearing loss had placed a severe strain on both, and I honestly do not know what I would be doing now, in either arena, without the implant. For me at least, the implant is nothing short of a miracle, and one which arrived in the very nick of time."

Not all implant surgeries are so successful. Beverly Biderman, an implant recipient and the author of an inspiring book, *Wired for Sound,* reports that a recent study evaluated sixty-one people six months after they had received implants. Their sentence comprehension, without lip cues, averaged 84 percent, but it ranged from 24 to 100 percent. I nevertheless reflected afterward on what implant surgery might have meant for Mother during her years of deafness (and frustration, embarrassment, and isolation). I realized that if I continue on her trajectory, I may not have to undergo her fate, and Carol may not need to endure and support a deaf spouse, as did my father. Indeed, in the 10 September 1999 issue of *Science,* Josef Rauschecker of the Georgetown University Medical Center reports on "a new generation of cochlear implants that combine multichannel technology with intelligent high-speed processors. These new devices permit word recognition rates of 80 to 100 percent (70 percent is sufficient to lead a phone conversation) and usually provide immediate success in adults who become deaf late in life. They are in demand by such individuals as well as by hearing parents of deaf children, and the costs of implant surgeries (about U.S. $40,000) are now covered by many U.S. health insurance companies and the British National Health Service."

The apparent effectiveness of the implants in conjunction with their high cost will surely pose an issue for medical ethics: How much is hearing worth? If cochlear-implant surgeries of the future reliably restore functional hearing, what should a person's remaining life expectancy be to warrant insurers and government health programs' footing the bill at $40,000 a person? We should bear in mind that all of us, ultimately, pay for such surgery—in reduced salaries (because our employers are funding the insurance bills) or through taxes. Should the surgery—and digital hearing aids (which are not covered by most plans)—be equally available to all, or only to the well-off? Before answering, we might consider this question: If at twenty we had no notion whether we would later suffer hearing loss, would we be willing to subsidize coverage for hearing aids and cochlear implants in case our number might come up on the devil's dice? If so, how much?

Better than Viagra? 17 FEBRUARY 2000

This year's omnipresent Viagra ads showing radiant older couples dancing or walking hand in hand could, with even greater reason, be recast as ads for hearing aids—or so the results of a new national survey suggest, as reported by Carolyn Holmes in the January/February 2000 issue of *Hearing Health.* The survey, involving 2,304 hard of hearing and 2,090 of their spouses, family members, or close friends, evaluated hearing loss and also assessed depression, anxiety, and social engagement. The striking result: whether experiencing mild or severe hearing loss, the hard of hearing were sadder and less socially engaged, and, when not using hearing aids, they felt others' irritation more (Figures 7.2–7.4).

The survey, undertaken for the National Council on the Aging, also asked those who had bought hearing aids whether they were experiencing emotional and social benefits. One-third reported improvements in their social life. Four in ten reported heightened self-confidence and better relationships with children and grandchildren. Fifty-six percent said "relationships at home" had improved.

Figure 7.2 Percentage Who Are Sad or Depressed (Two Weeks or More, Past Year)

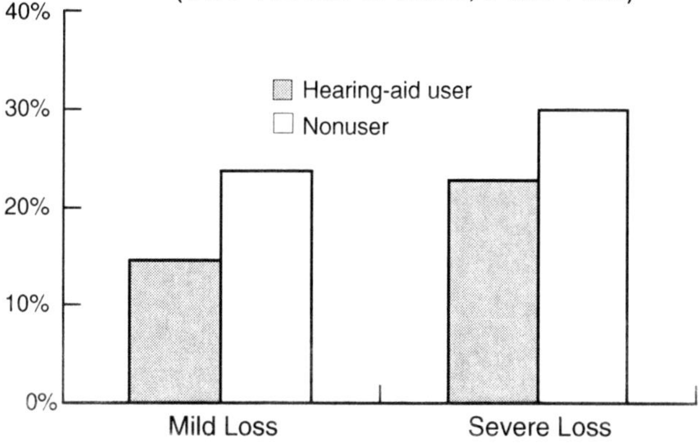

Figure 7.3 Percentage Who Participate Regularly in Social Activities

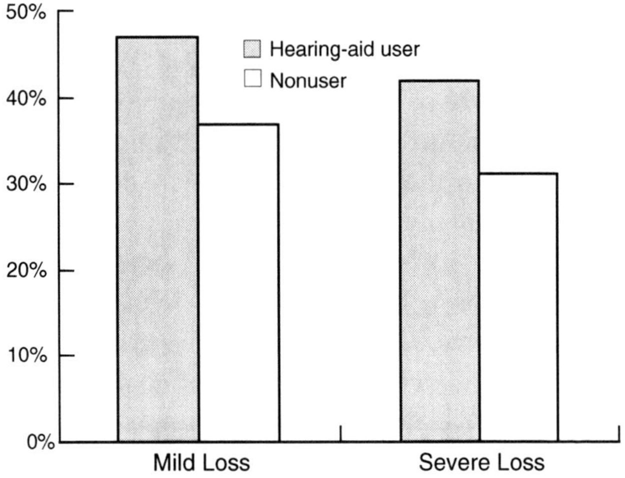

Figure 7.4 Percentage Who Say People Get Angry with Them for No Reason

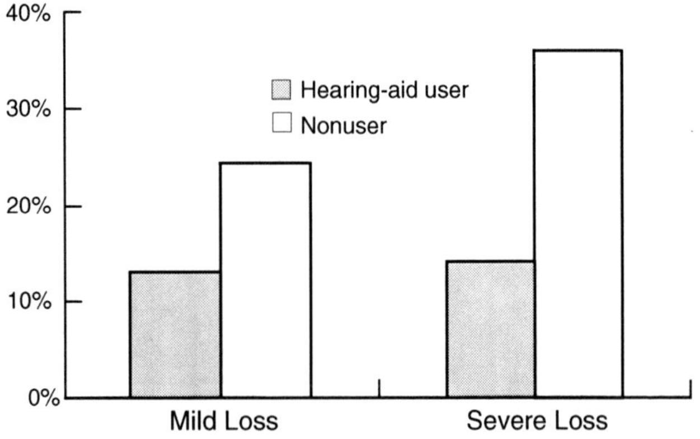

And what did their family members perceive? In each of these cases, they were even *more* likely to detect improvement. For example, 66 percent reported better relationships at home.

So why do most people with hearing loss not use hearing aids? Twenty percent said that wearing them "would make me feel old." More than half—55 percent—said "they are too expensive." More than two-thirds—69 percent—claimed, "My hearing isn't that bad," and virtually as many said, "I can get along without one." These, it seems, are the big three barriers to hearing aids: vanity, cost, and denial.

Blessed Are the Poor in Spirit 19 FEBRUARY 2000

Writing in the January–February 2000 issue of *Weavings*, spiritual director Judy Connato offers two interesting reflections on her hearing loss. First, she acknowledges her temptation, especially when fatigued, to view herself as a victim.

> After all, I reason, my life isn't easy. "They" should be more sensitive. "They" should speak more clearly, make their voices louder, remember that I can't hear when their backs are turned or lips are covered. When I slip into the role of victim, I endeavor to make my loss at least partially the responsibility of others. I have forgotten that this is *my* poverty, and therefore my responsibility to work out.

Second, she notes how awareness of her physical impoverishment helps her encounter her spiritual poverty, and then to sense God's grace.

> The hearing loss that is a component of my every interaction, whether I am listening to someone in the ministry of spiritual direction or sharing playful conversation with a friend, is an ever-present reminder that I am impoverished. Accepting this poverty, saying yes to it with as much free-

dom and love as I possibly can at that moment, allows me to live in the provisional present that God then transforms through grace. And I discover in these grace-filled moments one final, delightful paradox: it is my hearing loss that is my greatest hearing aid.

Epilogue

As we enter the new millennium, we are, more than usual, contemplating the future. In *The American Paradox: Spiritual Hunger in an Age of Plenty,* I reflected on our culture's recent past and envisioned its future. Now I do so for my own.

As Carol and I look at our lengthening past and shortening future, as we observe our own aging and the aging and death of our parents, we reflect on the sadness of the inevitable life cycle. We are born. We live—slowly, at first, it seems, then more rapidly, at least when we look back on it—and we die.

Facing the terror of our mortality, being aware of life's fragility and impermanence, does, however, make the present moment more precious. Facing death, rather than denying it, prepares us to celebrate life. Those, like my brother Jim, who have stared death in the face, know best how to cherish each remaining day. As a person oriented toward the future, I periodically remind myself of Pascal's remark that too often we live as if the past and present were merely our means to the future. "So we never live, but we hope to live—and as we are always preparing to be happy, it is inevitable we should never be so." With age, it becomes a little easier to treasure present pleasures—the cup of tea shared with a friend, the joy of a letter, the contentment of snuggling and talking after the lights are out.

As these simple pleasures suggest, one of the major roots of personal well-being is the enjoyment of close, enduring, supportive relationships. We all have what some social psychologists call a "need to belong." The human creature is, as Aristotle said, "the social animal." We are people who need people. We become human in relationships with others—an idea first expressed in the Old Testament creation story ("It is not good that the man should be alone"). We live not as solitary beings but in family groups that are organized into larger social systems. Deprived of natural social bonds, people will re-create them by forming clubs, gangs, and support groups. Anxiety, jealousy, loneliness, and guilt all stem from a threat to or disruption in our sense of belonging. Asked, "What is necessary for your happiness?" or "What is it that makes your life meaningful?" most people mention—before anything else—satisfying close relationships with family, friends, or romantic partners. As C. S. Lewis said, "The sun looks down on nothing half so good as a household laughing together over a meal."

It has been shown repeatedly that people with a network of intimate friends enjoy greater health, happiness, and longevity. In surveys of 35 thousand adults since 1972 by the University of Chicago's National Opinion Research Center, only 24 percent of never-married adults claimed to be "very happy," but 40 percent of married people did. Small wonder that hearing loss—a real impediment to close relationships—can prove so frustrating.

For now, my close relationships remain wonderfully significant. But knowing that hearing loss can be socially isolating, I often wonder, Will these relationships and life in general still be satisfying during retirement? How will I cope as the hearing loss progresses and the world becomes quieter? How will I feel about being unable to talk to friends on the phone, interact with uncomprehending strangers, or enjoy music? Will I need to curtail my travel and speaking engagements? Perhaps deafness will make my life, as one deaf person described it, like living inside a glass jar and seeing but not hearing others who are outside the jar.

New digital technology has offset my hearing loss during the last several years. Perhaps future technologies, combined with medical advances in hair-cell regeneration and stem-cell transplantation, will keep pace with my sensory decline. If not, perhaps a cochlear implant will renew my hearing. If, however, I progress from sound to silence, I surely will regret the loss. I will remember wistfully the symphony of sound I once knew. No doubt I will be in a better position to appreciate Helen Keller's statement that she "found deafness to be a much greater handicap than blindness. . . . Blindness cuts people off from things," she observed. "Deafness cuts people off from people."

But I reassure myself: I would discover new joys, and maybe even find some good within the misfortune. How fortunate I am that I love to read, think, and write—activities that deafness does not hamper and may even enhance. Henry Kisor, in his memoir of deafness, also reported feeling fortunate:

"Are you happy?" I was asked not long ago by someone who works in the world of the deaf.

I? I who have a loving spouse, two bright and strapping sons, a decent income, respect in my profession, a house in a pleasant suburb, and a host of good friends?

"Of course I am!" I all but shouted, exasperatedly throwing my hands into the air. I'm as happy as any other person whom life has nourished from a mixed plate of blessings and curses.

Although I wish my hearing were acute, the possibility of severe hearing loss neither frightens nor depresses me. Without deluding myself that the other benefits will compensate for sensory disability, I am optimistic that I will adapt, that I will develop new sensitivities, and that I will drink from other sources of lasting joy.

Appendix
Resources for the Hard of Hearing

Magazines on Hearing Loss

Hearing Health
P.O. Drawer V
Ingleside, TX 78362
www.hearinghealthmag.com

"Designed for people who experience any degree of hearing loss, tinnitus, or other ear disorder."

Hearing Loss
7910 Woodmont Avenue, Suite 1200
Bethesda, MD 20814
www.shhh.org/journal/hearloss.htm

"For people with hearing loss looking for the latest information on technology, products, services, national legislation, and coping, to help them live with their hearing loss."

Silent News
135 Gaither Dr., Suite F
Mount Laurel, NJ 08054–1710
www.silentnews.org

"World's most popular newspaper of deaf and hard of hearing people."

Assisted-Listening Resource Centers

Following is a partial list of companies with websites, catalogues, and stores offering different kinds of support to the hard of hearing.

Centrum Sound Systems

572 La Conner Dr.
Sunnyvale, CA 94087
members.aol.com/centrumweb

HARC Mercantile

P.O. Box 3055
Kalamazoo, MI 49003
www.harcmercantile.com

Harris Communications

15159 Technology Dr.
Eden Prairie, MN 55344
www.harriscomm.com

HearMore

42 Executive Blvd.
Farmingdale, NY 11735
www.hearmore.com

Hitec Group

8160 Madison Ave.
Burr Ridge, IL 60521
www.hitec.com

Potomac Technology

One Church St., Suite 101
Rockville, MD 20850–4158
www.potomactech.com

North American Nonprofit Organizations Serving the Hard of Hearing

Alexander Graham Bell Association for the Deaf

3417 Volta Place N.W.
Washington, DC 20007–2778
(202) 337–5220
www.agbell.org

Established "to empower persons who are hearing impaired." Advocates early identification of hearing loss and provides information and services to parents, educators, health professionals, and HOH adults

American Tinnitus Association
P.O. Box 5
Portland, OR 97207
(503) 248–9985
www.ata.org

Supports research and education concerning tinnitus.

Association of Late-Deafened Adults
1145 Westgate St., Suite #206
Oak Park, IL 60301
www.alda.org

"Serving the needs of late-deafened adults."

Better Hearing Institute
5021-B Backlick Rd.
Annandale, VA 22003
(703) 248–9985
www.betterhearing.org

The leading North American provider of free information about hearing.

Canadian Hard of Hearing
Association
2435 Holly Lane, Suite 205
Ottawa, Ontario, Canada K1V 7P2
(800) 263–8068
www.cyberus.ca/~chhanational

"Canada's only nation-wide Non-Profit Consumer Organization run by and for Hard of Hearing people."

Canadian Hearing Society
271 Spadina Rd.
Toronto, Ontario M5R 2V3
(416) 928–2504
www.chs.ca

"Provides services that enhance the independence of deaf, deafened, and hard of hearing people, and encourages prevention of hearing loss."

Hard of Hearing Advocates
245 Prospect St.
Framingham, MA 01701

(508) 875–8662
www.hohadvocates.org

Aims to "help hard of hearing (HOH) people by creating and implementing programs/solutions where HOH people have undue problems."

HEAR (Hearing Education and Awareness for Rockers)
P.O. Box 460847
San Francisco, CA 94146
(415) 773–9590
www.hearnet.com

"Dedicated to raising awareness of the real dangers of repeated exposure to excessive noise levels which can lead to permanent, and sometime debilitating, hearing loss and tinnitus. We're here for musicians, music fans, and anyone needing help with . . . hearing."

HIP (Hearing Is Priceless)
House Ear Institute
2100 West Third St., 5th Floor
Los Angeles, CA 90057
www.hei.org/htm/hipstart.htm

Aims "to change this perception by disseminating hearing health information to school students, entertainment industry and professionals, and the general public."

League for the Hard of
Hearing
71 West 23rd St.
New York, NY 10010–4162
(917) 305–7700
www.lhh.org

A New York City–based organization that seeks "to improve the quality of life for people with all degrees of hearing loss."

Self Help for Hard of Hearing People
7910 Woodmont Ave., Suite 1200
Bethesda, MD 20814
(301) 657–2248
www.shhh.org

The premier support organization for those who are hard of hearing. Provides publications and meetings.

Sight and Hearing Association
674 Transfer Rd.
St. Paul MN 55114-1402
(800) 992-0424
www.sightandhearing.org

"Dedicated to preventing the needless loss of vision and hearing through effective screening, education, and research."

International Nonprofit Organizations Serving the Hard of Hearing

(Member organizations of the International Federation of Hard of Hearing People)

Transnational Organizations

International Federation of Hard of Hearing People
P.O. Box 13
Abbots Langley
Hertfordshire, WD5 0RQ
United Kingdom
44-1923-264584
www.ifohh.org

"Consists of national associations of and for hard of hearing and late-deafened people, and parents' and professional organizations."

International Federation of Hard of Hearing Young People
Östra Långgatan 61
FIN-641 00
Kristinestad, Finland

Internationaler Verband für Schwerhörigen-Seelsorge e.V.
Krokusstrasse 1, D-48527
Nordhorn, Germany

Australia

Better Hearing Australia, Inc.
2 Gilbert St.
Gilberton, South Australia 5081
Australia
www.betterhearing.org.au

Austria

Österreichischer Bund für Schwerhörige, Spätertaubte, Tinnitus-Betroffene und Sprachbehinderte
61 Annenstrasse
A–8020 Graz, Austria

Belgium

Ligue Belge de la Surdité
avenue Henri de Brouckere 22
B–1160 Brussels, Belgium

Vereniging voor Hardhorenden "Onder Ons"
Haantjeslei 213
B–2018 Antwerp, Belgium

Croatia

Hrvatski savez gluhih i nagluhih
Croatian Association of the Deaf and Hard of Hearing
Palmoticeva 4
1000 Zagreb, Croatia

Czech Republic

Svaz neslysicich a nedoslychavyh v CR
Union of the Deaf and Hard of Hearing in the Czech Republic
Karlinske namesti 12
186 03 Praha 8
Czech Republic

Denmark

Landsforeningen for Bedre
Hørelse
Danish Association of the Hard of Hearing
Kloverprisvej 10B
DK–2650 Hvidovre, Denmark
www.lbh.dk

Estonia

Eesti Vaegkuuljate Uhing
Parnu mnt. 142
EE–0013 Tallinn, Estonia

Finland

Kuulonhuoltolitto r.y.,
Horselvardsforbundet
Finnish Federation of the Hard of Hearing
Ilkantie 4
FIN–00400 Helsinki, Finland
www.health.fi/kuulonhuoltolitto/english.html

France

Bureau de Coordination des Associations de Devenus Sourds et Malentendants
37 rue St.-Sébastien
F–75011 Paris, France

Germany

Deutscher Schwerhörigen-Bund e.V.
Schiffbauerdamm 13
D–10117 Berlin, Germany

Bundesgemeinschaft der Eltern und Freunde Hörgeschädigter
Pirolkamp 18
D–22397 Hamburg, Germany

Hungary

Siketek es Nagyothallok Orszagos Szevetsege
Hungarian National Association of the Deaf and Hard of Hearing
Benczur u. 21
1068 Budapest, Hungary

Ireland

Irish Hard of Hearing Association

35 N. Frederick St.
Dublin 1, Ireland
www.ihha.ie

Italy

Associazione nazionale per la lotta alla sordita e la tutela degli audiolesi

via Pestrino 6
I–30035 Mirano (VE), Italy
www.col.it/associ/audies/audies.html

Coordinamento Iniziative sui Problemi dei Sordi

via Alghero 1/17
I–16128 Genoa, Italy

Japan

Zenkoku Nancho-sha Renraku Kyogi-Kai Japan National Conference of the Hard of Hearing

MS Building Ichigayadai 2F, Ichigayadaimachi 14
Shinjyuku-ku 162
Tokyo, Japan

Kenya

Kenya Association of the Hard of Hearing

P.O. Box 10420
Nairobi, Kenya

Kuwait

Kuwait National Commission for Education, Science and Culture

P.O. Box 3266
13033 Safat, Kuwait

Netherlands

Federatie van Ouders van Slechthorende en Spraakgebrekkige Kinderen
P.O. Box 480
NL–3500 AL
Utrecht, Netherlands

Nederlandse Vereniging voor Slechthorenden
Kastordreef 3–5
3561 EJ
Utrecht, Netherlands
www.nvvs.nl

New Zealand

The Hearing Association
Top Floor, Community Services Building
The Strand
Takapuna, New Zealand
www.hearing.org.nz

Norway

Hörselhemmedes Landsforbund
Lilleakerveien 31a
0283 Oslo, Norway
www.hlf.no

Slovakia

Slovensky zvä z sluchovo postihnutch
Slovak Union of the Deaf and Hard of Hearing
Budatinska 59/a, 851 06 Bratislava, Slovakia
Correspondent: Mr. Milan Ruckay

Slovenia

Zdruzenje Naglusnih oseb Slovenije
Slovenian Association of Hard of Hearing People
Trg. Edvarda Kardelja 1, p.p. 185
5001, Nova Gorica, Slovenia
www.arctur.si/tisina

Zveza Gluhih Naglusnih Slovenija
Organisation of Deaf and Hard of Hearing Persons of Slovenia
Drenikova 24, SLO
61000 Ljubljana, Slovenia

Sweden

Hörselskadades Riksförbund
Swedish Association of the Hard of Hearing
Box 6605
S–11384, Stockholm, Sweden
www.hrf.se

Switzerland

Bund Schweizerischer Schwerhörigen Vereine
Schaffhauserstrasse 7
CH–8042
Zurich, Switzerland
www.bssv.ch

Société romande pour la lutte contre les effets de la surdité
avenue des Jordils 5
CH–1006 Lausanne, Switzerland

Turkey

Türkiye Isitme ve Konusma Rehabilitasyon Vakfi
Turkish Hearing and Speech Rehabilitation Foundation
P.K. 876, Karakoy
Istanbul, Turkey

United Kingdom

Hearing Concern
7–11 Armstrong Rd.
London W3 7JL
web.ukonline.co.uk/hearing.concern

Zambia

Zambia National Association of the Hearing Impaired
Hearing and Speech Centre/UTH
P/Bag RW 448X
Lusaka, Zambia

Index